"The greatest pleasure in life is doing what people say you cannot do" –

Walter Bagehot

Letitcia

Body Worship

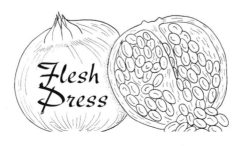

Flesh Press

First edition published 2004 by Flesh Press,
an imprint of Pomegranate Press
51 St Nicholas Lane, Lewes, Sussex BN7 2JZ
email: pomegranatepress@aol.com
website: pomegranate-press.co.uk

ISBN 0-9533493-8-1

British Library Cataloguing-in-Publication Data.
A catalogue record for this book is available from the British Library.

Printed by Cliffe Enterprise, 112 Malling Street, Lewes,
East Sussex BN7 2RJ
Telephone: 01273 483890

FOREPLAY

Write a book, they said . . . so I did
(even though they doubted my literary prowess)

My noon appointment strode up the stairs to my apartment bearing a beautiful bouquet of lilies and a bottle of vintage Moet. I had kept him waiting 15 minutes, and I apologised with the self-satisfied words: 'Sorry to keep you – I'm just finishing my book.'

'What book are you reading?' he replied.

Ha, bloody ha. Actually he was joking. You can always rely on a Yorkshireman to have a sense of humour.

Two days earlier, having bumped into 'filthy Simon', (named due to his sexual prowess), I was posed the question: 'Who's writing it for ya?'

Ha, bloody ha again.

My mate Harry asked one day: 'So watcha gonna call it, then?'

'*Quid pro quote.*'

'You're 'avin' a larf.'

'It works on many levels: quid – money; pro – prostitute; quote – talking.'

'Nobody understands, let alone bleedin' talks, Latin any more.'

'*Carpe Noctem*, then. Seize the night.'

'It's still Latin.'

'*The Real Goddess.*'

'Oi, oudya think you are, that domestic bird with the great tits?'

'*View From a Broad.*'

'Bette Midler used it.'

'*Ooker*'

'Wos that all abart?'

'*The Contented Lady.*'

'Sarnds like that bleedin' movie *The English Patient.*'

[Three weeks later]

'*Body Worship.*'

'Why didn't ya call it that to begin wiv, yer dopey car? Now let's go an' 'ave a swift 'alf!'

[Lights fade and we walk off into the sunset]

ACKNOWLEDGEMENTS

In the beginning was the word – Microsoft word, a world that was initially brought to my attention by David and Gordon, who resolved to drag me kicking and screaming into the arcane science of websites and computer technology. 'But I don't know how to turn it on,' I cried. They very patiently told me it would be an indispensable part of my life (like wanking). They were right. My gratitude to the following 'technical support team'.

Thank you, Mr Ken Paul, for purloining my very first piece of equipment, for setting it up and for responding to my pathetic cries for help when things went horribly wrong.

These sentiments are also for Mr. H. James Stocker, who would be 'back up' for when I had exhausted poor Kent with my demands. He valiantly saw off bugs and viruses (computer-wise) until we were overwhelmed by the sheer volume – the outome being yet another exhausted member of the team. A big thanks to Mr 'comfortable shoes' G., for guiding me in the right direction, especially when my first few chapters crashed and burned along with my 'pooter. To Doctor Tech, who miraculously retrieved my fledgling words from my defunct 'hard drive'.

Much gratitude to Mark 'the spit' (private joke), who configured the computer so that I might begin writing in the first place and inspired me to commit his magnificent presence into a few paragraphs. (Let's see if you can find them).

A huge hug to dear Noah, who by now has developed a nervous facial tic of paranoia whenever the phone rings lest it be me giving him reams of instructions for the design of either my book or my website. I work him hard and he delivers (usually) with a degree of excellence to which I have become accustomed.

To my 'main man' Carl, a tongue-less kiss for solving the distribution and sales problem, and also for putting the hilarious idea into my mind (which was burst forth in *his*) that everyone buying 50 books should receive a personalised blow-up Letitcia doll. What a sense of humour . . .

A raised glass to Harry, who keeps trying to drill into me that 'life is a constant struggle between form and content', sagely asserting that there is too much of one and lamentable sod all of the other. When these ripe pearls of wisdom are spoken in the broadest of 'yer 'avin' a larf' Essex wideboy the only thing one can do is giggle uncontrollably.

Commiserations to the 'other halves': D. Harrison, Richard, Lydia, Will and Tracy for having to concede defeat in keeping the evening repast of edible quality due to my neediness of their partners' valuable time for their particular area of expertise and the fact that I think the entire universe revolves around me, me, me.

Many thanks to David Arscott, for stoically entering 'a world less travelled' (I think) and for embracing it rather than dismissing it judgementally out of hand. The convoluted journey of book publishing has been made much easier and clearer than I ever thought possible – and his missus makes a right nice cuppa.

To Julie, many thanks for having the wisdom to tell the difference between the profession and the person and for graciously giving me advice and support.

Finally to my family, with whom I am blessed. I am provided with unconditional love and support for whatever I want to do (since trying to talk me out of it would be futile). I can be what I want to be and do what I want to do without fear or favour. Not many people can say that.

Let's read on, Macduff, and see what I've been up to for the last decade or so . . .

CONTENTS

Jostling for pole position — 13

The juxtaposition of men, sex and their cars and parking arrangments – or, in some cases, doggy and wheelchair arrangements.

The things you see when you haven't got a gun — 19

Illuminating experiences of what lurks beneath men's trousers. By one who's in a prime situation to know.

Pulchritude v Bushpig Central — 23

Dispels the myth that young gorgeous women make the best sex workers. Personal anecdotes to prove such.

Merchantable quality — 27

Dispels a further myth – that non-workers are cleaner in their personal hygiene than sex works. Statistics and personal experience to support this fact.

Well, cover me in chocolate and throw me to the lesbians! — 31

The most frustrating account of trying to find quality in the sex-for-sale market. My personal account of trying to find a male escort.

Six degrees of gravy — 39

The premise of six degrees of separation where sex is concerned, with personal anecdotes.

Turgid conscience 45

Men: their inherent disloyalty and infidelity. Social comment based on personal experiences.

Revving it up 51

Sex and religion: the hypocrisy that I have seen with my own eyes, with reference to a newspaper article previously published about a vicar and me.

Drop the AK 47 55

A discourse of whimsy about making love and not war. A flight of fancy based upon the fact that there is so much hatred in the world.

Slap my thigh and ride in on the wave 60

Posing the question: do men like big women? Personal experiences and anecdotes.

Don't panic, Mr Mainwaring! 65

Hilarious examples of when jobs go horribly wrong.

Going down, Down Under 73

What it's like to work in Australia, and my interpretation of how Aussie men perform in bed.

Sick puppies 80

Dealing with the most popular question ever asked: what's the kinkiest shit you've ever done. My fascinating and disgusting answer.

Travels with my c(a)unt: Part 1 90

Travelling in South-east Asia, buying a male prostitute in Thailand and various sexual encounters along the way.

Contents

Travels with my c(a)unt: Part 2   101
Beach boy gigolos in Malaysia; nuances arising from
their religion and culture; their hypocrisy regarding sex
with white women.

**Come on baby, light my fire (or at least
make me smoulder)**   111
The first man to give me an orgasm. Differing sexual
practices among diverse ethnic backgrounds.

Entente cordiale (Kofi, we need you)   119
Perceived mistrust between black and white people,
and preconceptions against prostitutes.

Rump wrangling (the hard yard)   125
Dispels the myth of clear delineation between
gay/straight and the complications therein.

Charging like a wounded bull   132
Setting one's price in a world with no RRP.

Charity chuffs   137
Women who charge and amateurs who give it away.

Aroma coma   143
What to do with clients who need a good tub-up.

Date bait   148
Looking for a companion via newspaper dating services.
Personal experiences.

Hoochie momma   153
What happens when you fall for a punter.

Stitch in time   157

The amount of plastic surgery that neurotic working girls have done in an effort to stay attractive to their clientele.

Taking it in the mouth for cash   160

How sexual practices changed when AIDS reared its ugly head in Australia.

Shy and retiring   164

What happens when I retire: punters' attitude.

Cult of personality   168

Preying on the weak. The perceived notion that sex workers need saving from themselves.

Boys with toys   175

Men and sex aids – like kids in a sweet shop.

You take the high road and I'll take the low road – but how low can you go?   179

Body parts that never get touched.

Boring an arsehole in a wooden horse   182

Why I don't do tedious.

Cum on, feel the noise   188

Aural sex, and the imaginative scenes a girl has to create to satisfy a range of sexual pleasures.

The rear end   192

Jostling for Pole Position

The New York lesbian collective SCUM asserted that a man had only one thing on his mind. They stated that he would crawl on his belly through a river of viscous snot and vomit, to reach a welcoming vagina. Not true. There are really only two things that matter in the world to men, and anything else pales into insignificance.

World War Three may be declared, famine, plague and pestilence may sweep the four corners of the globe, civilizations may crumble and governments may be overturned, but the overriding questions on every man's lips are: 'Can I get a suck without a condom?' and 'What's the parking like round there?'. Strangely, both requests are often asked in the same sentence.

I swear if they could drive their car up the stairs they would. I have housed myriad skateboards and mountain bikes (some would say, due to the young age of my patrons, 'You mean tricycles, surely?') in my vestibule. They are reticent to leave their favoured mode of transport out of their sight.

If a man is thinking of his car while getting laid I wonder if the spark plugs bristle in sexual sympathy and the big end swells while the driver is unavoidably detained. And if man and car are so inextricably linked, why doesn't the horn blare out and the hazard lights blink when the dirty deed is done?

To be able to leap from libido to the practicalities of life is quite curious. Maybe it's a 'man and his car' thing with a bit of automotive penile extension thrown in. Consider the following conversation:

'Yeah hi, Letitcia! Where's the best place to park my car?'

'Side of the road works for most people, pal.'

'Ah, very funny. Seriously, is it off-street parking or vouchers?'

'Sorry, I don't own a car – you're on your own there. You just park your car and I'll do the rest, ok?'

'In that case I'll leave it, thanks. Don't want another ticket.'

Once, a young virgin (the lovely Ryan who was all of sweet 16, at least that's what it claimed on his bus pass) stated that had I been 300 yards further along the road he would probably have considered option two, because it would have been too far from his bus stop. *This is a seminal moment in a young man's life and he's belly-aching about marginal travel arrangements!* Bad habits start real early.

Young Ryan was extremely industrious regarding money, or shall we say *lack thereof*. He had hit upon an ingenious way to raise the necessary capital to prompt me into action. Quite apart from his pre-school paper round and his pocket money, he cajoled and begged (without so much as a smidgeon of embarrassment) to be allowed to rub my back, feet, and anything else I needed rubbing for that matter, in return for being allowed to stay longer than the sum total of his measly stipend.

The Chinese aristocracy used to send their young men to 'professionals' to give them the best possible sexual start in life. If the British government ever gets its head round the fact that not only *politicians* patronise hookers, then I would certainly put my name forward as the 'main man' were an academy of erotic excellence to be the recipient of lottery handouts.

As for young, dumb, and full of so much come that he could barely navigate the stairs (so large was his ardour), I decided fresh-faced Ryan should be taught the lesson that if something is *too* accessible you will not feel the supreme pleasure, and goaded him to try and match the going rate which the grown-ups paid. He did not disappoint, bless him.

It transpired that any new piece of apparel his parents bought for him would be taken back to the original shop on the pretext of whatever lie a pubescent lad with raging hormones (and hard on) could muster. His parents couldn't understand his lack of clothes when they kept doling out money for Nike-this and Calvin Klein-that.

It is with pride that I received *department store vouchers* to supplement paying for his sexual education. (Some bright spark tried to offer me B&Q vouchers the other day, but a woman has her pride – plus my fingers are erotic, not green.)

I received both him and the vouchers many times before his parents decided to relocate. (Had they known of his activities after school and before his steak and kidney pud I have a sneaky suspicion they would have emigrated to Antarctica to cool his lust).

He hitch-hiked a few times to maintain contact and a fabulous sex life with yours truly, but the distance proved too far – and besides, his clothes were getting threadbare.

Luckily (for him) he had managed to saunter the extra few yards for his very first schoolboy fumble, thereby starting his sexual experiences at the very top – *thus* ensuring that he would require extensive psycho/sexual counselling for the rest of his natural born. On such small things moments of great historical importance can hinge.

Man's parking dilemma: what a pain in the neck! I have to turn into the ultimate 'flexible friend'. So flexible, in fact, that it's a triple somersault with a double twist (a compulsory 9.8 score, Olympics wise). My seafront apartment, which is the customer's demi-monde and haven from the heaving unforgiving world, is transformed into a WW2 Battle of Britain-esque ops room. Frantic calls to various accommodating, car space-owning neighbours ensues with enquiries about ETA or departure of all interested parties. Even then this flurry of activity is not enough.

'Letitcia, the space isn't big enough for my car. It's the latest Merc. Are you sure I can't put it the other side?'

Exasperation and an instant migraine rears its head.

The end result being that I need a cup of tea, an aspirin and a power nap due to exhaustion, and *not* a two hour session of rumpy pumpy with an anally retentive Mercedes-driving dude. All you need to *completely* stuff the whole scenario is a white van man to arrive on scheduled maintenance work, and, *voilà*: mayhem.

I had occasion to work in Australia's premier massage parlour. The establishment (like the employees) used both front and back entrances. Customers would routinely rock up with 'man's best friend' (no, not an air tight alibi). Pooches of varying sizes and temperament would be dragged out by 'Mr Gagging-For-It-But-Need-Excuse-To-Leave-The-House'. The leash would be proffered to Pete, the maintenance man at the rear entrance, along with a screwed up five-dollar bill and that old chestnut, 'Back in a mo, mate, got a bit of growling at the badger to do'. (To the uninitiated that's *cunnilingus*.)

Leaving Pete with a yapping mutt was not conducive to the customers already inside, who were already engaging in reaching 'the vinegar stroke', so he would drag the offending doggie off for a walk. Word got round that we offered this particular service, and a familiar and yet hilarious sight was Pete grappling with various breeds of the canine persuasion (not unlike the concierges of New York) around the leafy suburbs of Surrey Hills, Sydney. This earned him the soubriquet 'Doggie Pete', thereby making the ladies think he was unoriginal in bed.

A postscript to this scenario is the fact that once the customer had both his cock and mind blown he would invariably exit via the *front* door, leaving the poor creature behind. (I am not making this up.)

Then there was the dash for the 'best waiting room'. I had two regular patrons who had a propensity for being 'the first cab off the rank'. I don't know why men insist on this quaint positioning – it's not as if anyone is receiving 'sloppy seconds'. We have moved on a long way from a bowl of grey disinfected water and an even greyer flannel being dragged across our 'bits'. My regulars both used to arrive one hour before their allotted time. The parlour didn't actually take appointments, but they had to make an exception in my case, such was the demand. Unfortunately for me, they both used to choose the same day (Sunday at seven in the morning), which meant that I had two men hot-to-trot at six a.m. Why a man would think he could get the best out of a woman at this ungodly hour is beyond my female powers of comprehension.

They both would be upset at *a*) having to be kept waiting, *b*) not snaring the best waiting room. They both upped the ante and started to arrive so early I was getting up at *three* in the morning to cover the illusion that one or t'other was my one and only start of the day. Very frustrating, and all the more aggravating, by virtue of the fact that when they both got fed up with what they thought was a cavalier attitude to their custom, they *both changed their day*. Yep, you guessed it. Saturday was now my appointed day of dissemblance. In Formula 1 parlance, they didn't want any other driver in the race: they wanted to be the 'safety car'.

The aforementioned front door was at street level and just peachy for wheelchair access. And so, from time to time, we would entertain vanloads of severely horny, yet equally severely disabled, young men. We had to make sure the entire ground floor was vacant, since the logistics of lifting our charges up and down the spindly staircase of the grand town houses (three knocked into one) would have been unfeasible – and might have resulted in the number of 'disabled' on the premises exceeding some bullshit fire and safety regulation.

How stoic of the carers to facilitate a right royal 'seeing to' for the 'wheelies' and to forego one themselves. Afterwards a few of us would escort them onto the street. They looked like Rag, Tag and Bobtail, some in their 'sweet chariots', some piggy-backed by the carers, and some (though rather unsteadily) under their own steam. To looks of astonished passers by, we would claim, 'Youse should've seen 'em three hours ago, mate! Strapping rugger buggers every one of 'em!'

Had the 'B' division of the city's fire department been visiting in their fire engine (as was their wont) we would have had the trifecta of surrealism at the best little whorehouse in the Antipodes.

Funnily enough, it didn't have a car park . . .

The Things You See When You Haven't Got a Gun

I once ventured to an abysmal Saturday night party in Brighton and pulled a not altogether unattractive young man from Holland. I was at my most charming and witty, and he was coerced into a taxi (despite protestations of needing to catch flights to foreign parts the next day).

Up the stairs. . . in my apartment . . . through to the boudoir . . . keep on coming baby . . . just put one step in front of the other and the body will follow . . .

Finally, splayed on my futon, I couldn't understand his reluctance to remove his socks, shoes and chinos. Therefore I did the dutiful handmaiden/geisha bit – one shoe; one sock; god this boy could kiss; next shoe – arrrrghhh, its bionic man himself! A *weird* Teflon foot confronted madame.

I surreptitiously began stroking his leg to see how far this novel contraption extended. Phew! Just half the foot, fortunately. Nothing was mentioned by either party (such an Anglo-Saxon thing to do). It did make me realise though that men with some physical disfigurement are *animals* in the sack.

Reel back ten years earlier to the magnificent spa room in Sydney's finest sin emporium. On my return to the room, the strapping Aussie rules player who had minutes before been left to freshen up was almost literally half the man he was. Well, okay, I'm embellishing here but *an entire leg was casually leaning against the shower cubicle.*

Same thing as with Mr Teflon. Nothing was mentioned, and I obliged him with the standard blow-job which all 'cobbers' seem to love. Now, I'm no doctor but I couldn't work out why the more I sucked the higher the 'stump' rose, until I lost my concentration entirely due to this involuntary reaction. Rising to the occasion is all fine and dandy, but in this case it was the wrong body part.

Another brothel, another freak show lurking in the trousers. Mr. Yamamoto, interpreter and leader of the group of hopeful customers, was in earnest discussion with our head supervisor. He was looking a little less inscrutable, and the conversation was becoming more heated, as the minutes wore on – the reason being that his charge of Japanese and Korean businessmen had some aberration within their Y-fronts and were worried how we'd react.

The ladies reasoned that 'it was nothing we hadn't seen before', and we led them to the rooms chuckling that we would probably find Lord Lucan or even Shergar the racehorse himself.

I forget who screamed first, but we girls all reconvened outside on the stairs to swap notes.

'How many has yours got, then?'

'Looks like about seven, but to tell you the truth it made me feel like chundering so I stopped counting.'

'Well it might actually be nice once we get in the saddle.'

It seems that there is an arcane tradition among certain Japanese/Korean fisherman which demands that valuable *black sea pearls* are somehow inserted under the foreskin, creating the appearance of the ugliest dick you have ever squared up to in your life.

Whether this is done to convey monetary status, or for sexual pleasure (and trust me on this one it does *not*) we never found out, since we had embarrassed our yellow perils and great face was lost all round.

It gives a whole new meaning to the ad phrase 'suck a fisherman's friend'.

Three a.m. and the graveyard shift is suffering from exhaustion. A likely lad wanders in and chooses me.

'Hey, youse look like you're a good root,' he opined.

'Looks like you're about to find out big boy,' I replied.

Sunny Jim drops his trousers to reveal (I am not making this up) a semen-filled condom clinging to his manhood.

'Looks like you've come already,' I said.

Without one ounce of embarrassment he smiled and jeered: 'Shit, that was an hour ago. You mean she didn't take it off?'

As I shook my head he continued: 'Yeah, well that what youse get for goin' with them street sheilas.'

How can one be angry at a complete drongo? We girlies scrub teeth and tongue, floss and rinse, gargle and suspend consumption of all food for hours before a dental appointment. But the Lesser-spotted Great Aussie Ocker does no prep work for working ladies and smiles in the face of such embarrassment. Why do I actually believe they wipe their dicks on the bedroom curtains?

When my playful mood takes over I often josh my patrons that I am not a tart but both a learned anthropologist and a bona fide stooge for a conglomerate of underwear companies. Who is better placed to discover the male punter's dark dank secret hidden beneath his trousers?

'Christmas present then?' I enquire when confronted with eye-watering dynarod florescent orange and lime-green golfing shorts.

Many punters represent M&S, Next and/or Tie Rack, and approximately 3 per cent wear Y-fronts. (And some are none too clean I can tell you, *what is wrong with these people?*). The more adventurous strike a pose in Klein and Ralph Lauren and, thank Christ ,I have only encountered a few leather/leopard print, excruciatingly nasty G-strings on the most incongruous of old swingers (Barf).

My personal favourite was a dude who was obsessed by the glam/rock band KISS. He had a slinky pair of boxers printed with images of the band. Must be nice to have Gene Simmon's tongue rubbing against your bell-end.

Bringing up the rear (if you will pardon the expression) is Master of the Universe, commuter of the 7.17 London-Brighton stockbroker train. Tristan has booked an hour appointment and phones ahead to say: 'Cannot wait to see you'.

'Why, thanks,' I reply.

'No, I really can't wait to see you,' he whines.

All is revealed upon arrival. Disrobing his Turnbull and Asser bespoke shirt, complete with diamond cufflinks, designer suit and exquisite hand-made shoes he finally reveals the object of his discomfort – *a stainless steel custom-made butt plug plus testicle and penile restrainer.*

Seems he finds the ultimate pleasure in trading millions on the stock exchange while being in dire need from both front and back botty.

As if life isn't hard enough!

Pulchritude

v

Bushpig Central

Bumped into an acquaintance the other day, and being in a frightful hurry I wailed in passing, 'Can't stop, have incoming wounded to sort' – this being a euphemism for 'Am up to my tits in appointments'. His indelicate rejoinder was 'Jesus, if *you're* getting laid there's hope for all of us.'

A bitchy barb? Most certainly! An element of truth? Mmm, that's a tricky one.

The inference was (I assume) that since I'm a peri-menopausal woman of a certain age in this world of facelifts, dieting and image obsession, it defied credulity that anybody would want to bed me – let alone pay. Some saddo actually signed my website guest book once with the words: 'Too expensive for me baby. I know antiques are dear, but they still have to be in good shape.' How I laughed at that one.

How can one be subjective about beauty if it's your own? (I have been young and beautiful, but not necessarily at the same time.) Are gorgeous women the most successful sex workers?

Its 7pm: seconds out, round one for the evening shift in Victoria Street, Sydney. The dressing room is drenched in a haze of hair spray, deodorant and fine perfume. The nails are painted, the hair coiffed, breasts shown to their utmost advantage. Legs are waxed and the Bermuda triangle, or 'map of Tasmania' as it's called, is buffed to meet the most stringent scrutiny.

Estee Lauder, the cosmetic mogul, proclaimed that there was no such thing as ugly women, only those that didn't care or those who truly believed they were unattractive. And then there was *Nana Banana* . . .

She earned her moniker due to the fact she bore more than a passing resemblance to the Greek singer Nana Mouskouri, and her nose made Concorde look the size of a hanglider. Friends, she was 'ugly as a hat full of arseholes'. The milk bottle glasses and greasy hair, together with pigeon chest and flat bottom, completed what was probably one of the most inclement looking females in the universe. Yet Nana was *always* busy. Men flocked to worship at the altar of this physically-challenged woman.

A male friend explained: 'They think they're going to get the best shag of their life because she'll try harder.'

'You mean like a goat being fucked at the edge of a cliff – it pushes back?' I replied.

'Something like that. She must have got the job somehow. Don't you sheilas all get to do a try-out with the owner?'

I smiled benevolently at this deluded soul, 'No,' I sighed, 'it doesn't work like that.' (Sorry to disabuse you of *that* notion lads.)

Even the delectable Mr. Courvoisier (so named because he was a fancy licker) fell for her dubious charms.

'How long's he been with her?' my co-workers asked.

'An hour and a half,' I replied through gritted teeth.

'But he *never* stays for longer than half,' she spat.

'Well, she must have something that we don't,' I said.

'Yeah, right – frigging pimples and halitosis,' was her sarcastic reply.

Mr C's visit to Nana annoyed us all so much because we looked forward to being the lucky recipient of his feather-like tongue and deft touch. This man had turned love-making into an art form. He had a 100 per cent success rate with *every one of the girls.*

There were no favourites: he serviced us all with the same mind-blowing result. He took great pride in his endeavours as if it was a test that he must pass. So either Nana was being a bit slow out of the orgasmic starting block or (as some wag reasoned) he had his head heaving down the toilet bowl.

Then the JFC. buzzer rang.

Let me explain. We had a quirky tradition at the Surrey Hill emporium whereby when an employee achieved orgasm there was a secret buzzer thoughtfully provided to register the fact in the main reception area, and since the climax was generally accompanied by howls of 'Jesus Fucking Christ!' it earned that particular acronym.

We never got to the bottom of her popularity, but we reasoned that since she was *always* busy she had to be doing something right. God knows, I have seen international superstars (whose wives were mega-gorgeous) spend days with a complete 'bow wow'. The adage of men always wanting something different was time and again starkly illustrated. Conversely, some of the most stunning girls were the least successful due, one assumes, to the fact that they adopted that timeworn 'I am so attractive you should be grateful' attitude.

There is a famous French movie called (if memory serves me correctly) 'Too beautiful for you' in which a man embarks on an affair with a plain woman in stark contrast to his elegant ravishing wife – the subtext being that his missus was cold and unresponsive while his lover was shit-hot between the sheets.

This is something that women fail to realize: it doesn't matter how perfect your features are, it doesn't matter what weight you are or what breast size you are. If you can't hold your mate's attention sexually, and if you aren't continually being inventive and exploring areas of sensuality or eroticism, your looks alone will not save the day.

Only the other day, a patron imparted to me advice his father had given him at the age of *twelve*: 'Son, when you first go out and meet women, remember this – *Would you rather have an ugly fuck or a posh wank?*'

If I may paraphrase that music colossus Kid Rock: 'If it looks good you'll see it . . . if its marketed right you'll buy it . . . but if its real you'll *feel* it.'

So yes, maybe there *is* hope for all of us.

Merchantable Quality

On a girlie evening out in the badlands and fleshpots that Sydney has to offer in abundance, we, the ladies of Victoria Street, decided to do a bit of prossie bonding to celebrate a workmate's birthday. All went swimmingly until a visit to the toilet proved to be an insult too far.

A lady going about her ablutions muttered under her breath (yet loud enough for her intended recipients to hear) the unoriginal phrase: 'Bloody whores!' One can always rely upon an Aussie to have a mouth like the proverbial dunny. Dayl-lin our little pocket rocket from the Philippines (fuelled by copious amounts of drink, drugs and rock and roll) launched an attack which even Mr Jean Claude Van Damme would have applauded.

As she bashed the foul-mouthed interloper against the cistern, Robbie, the most verbose of our group sneered, 'at least we're not syphilitic, spit-fuck *charity moles!*'

Erroneous concept – all working ladies are disease-ridden harridans while all non-workers are pure as driven slush.

Excuse me. The judge's decision is final, the votes are in and these are our findings . . .

According to statistics from both pre- and ante-natal clinics in Australia a staggering 80 per cent of 'Let me take your shoes off and your tea's on the table' ideal Stepford wives are raddled with some STD or other. *Fact!* For some reason these censorious ladies think that 20 acts of unprotected sex in the name of fun is more hygienic and safer than 2,000 acts of *safe* sex performed while making financial whoopee.

Office workers getting jiggy with it on a regular basis would never consider popping along to the local clap clinic. Working girls in Australia (or at least those employed at top notch brothels) had to pay for this privilege.

'Hey doc,' I would say. 'Do ya think you can get that lamp a bit closer. My minge isn't on fire yet.'

Without a certificate of pristine health one couldn't work anywhere in the premier brothels of Australia. We took no delight in informing customers (male and female) that *their* nether regions needed medical attention. And we had to dispense this information fairly often. The rule in most up-market establishments was that the customer had to pass the 'corona physical' before he could proceed with the 'horizontal mambo'. We were trained to within a P of a PhD in gynaecological health.

This superior knowledge got interesting when boyfriends or husbands dragged their (unwilling) partners along for (yawn) a spot of menage a trois. It's bad enough that she doesn't want to be there; it's even worse that the man proceeds *almost completely* to ignore his partner when fresh meat is suddenly available. But the real kick in the pants is to tell a man that he can't be entertained because his lover is a walking STD. You've never truly seen a 'domestic' until you've rejected the 'Wendy house' of a sexually rapacious mate.

'Well, if I've got something you must as well,' she'll say to deflated hubby.

'How do I know its anything to do with me?' he will neatly counter, in the time-honoured tradition of apportioning blame

'How do I know you haven't been screwing around?'

You get the picture! Often the argument can be heard from miles away, and the worst thing is they can't even kiss and make up since she's (according to the magnified lamp and speculum) poxed up.

One couple that did scrape under the medical criteria was a Greek duo who were made for one another: they both had similar moustaches. The husband explained that he merely wanted to watch (how original) me make love to his wife, who was glowering in a decidedly unfriendly fashion. A more unappetising prospect would have been hard to find.

She was signalling that if I so much as went anywhere near Mr Lover Man my meat would be minced mousakka-style. She could stun a rhino from a thousand paces.

When feigned enthusiasm meets stubborn resistance the result is not pretty. I made a professional stab at executing an 'unpalatable manoeuvre', if you get my drift, but found the whole procedure disconcerting because instead of lying back and luxuriating in my touch she was have having a semi-row with Mr Zorba regarding, one assumes, the fact that he had the temerity to look at me (much less touch me).

He thankfully engaged in the proceedings and was interactive with the top half of his dearly beloved. I laboured on in the lower decks of the 'good ship uninterested' and pausing mid-effort saw *this stream of urine spurting over my bed*. My look of horror was countered by the husband's look of extreme satisfaction.

'See how my woman comes,' he crowed.

'Mate,' I replied, 'she's just pissed herself.'

A little word in your shell-like, you would-be Lotharios. When you're jiggling your digits, piston engine-like in a woman's vagina they will piss. *Read my lips*. It's an involuntary golden shower and not hoochie-momma mist.

So to the uneducated and bigoted general public (and you don't know who you are, because you are mistakenly languishing in your imagined cleanliness and your immoral high ground) *take note*: condoms are used to protect *us* from *you*, rather the reverse.

On a lighter note, a young sheep-sheerer from Queensland once shuffled penguin style to the 'checking lamp' to say 'Jeez, didn't know you charged by the inch.'

I started to check him, but tried not to be too robust as he looked ready to blow.

'You jerkin' me off before we start?' he exclaimed.

I explained the clinical procedure and he joked: 'All the sheep on our farm are Bonza, you'll not find anything wrong with *me*.'

I say 'joked', loosely. Another statistic, (though I don't quite know how they did the market survey), is that at some point in time a staggering 75 percent of jackaroos/farmhands, have had intimate relations with one or more of the livestock to hand.

He surveyed the opulent room and said: 'My dad told me not to go outside the 5k rule but it looks worth it to me'.

'Explain,' I prompted, intrigued.

'Youse never walk a Sheila more than five kilometres from the local dance hall, or if it's by horseback no journey that takes more than five minutes. Then, if you're real desperate, it's the five-case rule – five cases of beer to help you forget what a bushpig she is.

Long live education.

Well, Cover Me in Chocolate and Throw Me to the Lesbians!

The New Year loomed and I suddenly experienced an epiphany. I would hire a male escort. I would 'come' as the old year went. How hard could it be? Here is a salutary tale.

Lulled into my emboldened state of misplaced equality, I began my quest. Here, there and indeed everywhere no hunka burnin' love was safe from my clutches. I was on a mission. I would stalk him with the cunning and guile of the she-predator.

Surfing – clicking and double-clicking my way around sites which (erroneously) proclaimed that women could, indeed, indulge themselves with a *heterosexual* man of their dreams, if their ardour was strong enough and their wallet deep enough – I dove into a vat of men who all bore the same physical characteristics. Eighty per cent of these would-be gigolos whose posted 'photos' of themselves on the internet sported a blob of Vaseline masquerading as their visage. The remainder of them? Ahem! Well, they just splayed their tackle much as a butcher would display prime steaks on a slab of marble.

A few blind alleys and myriad gay sites later *I hit pay dirt.* London men for women – mmm, I could lick a truckload of whipped cream off those suckers with no problem whatsoever. This is where things came unstuck.

Pay attention ladies: it will save you endless phone calls, general gnashing of teeth and a *shit* load of money

'Hi, I'd love to book an escort and I like the look of A B & C. What's the SP?'

Lena the head honcho replies: 'I'll email or text them and get right back to you.'

Three days later, still no reply. I ask: 'Any news'?

'A is filming in Milan, B hasn't got back to me and C is on a modelling assignment it Bratislava.'

'Any chance of them being in England by the New Year?'

'Hard to say,' she replied 'but we do have D available'

Ten calls later, D rings for an initial briefing. The trouble was that the attractive young man sporting baby-oiled abs and an enigmatic stare *could not string a sentence together.* We ladies are funny creatures. We desire the whole package (no pun intended) – especially if it's charging £250 per hour.

Back to looking for Mr Goodbar.

Another week rolls by and model E rings to ask when I require his (or anybody else's) services. When I requested the weekend he baldly stated in the most hilarious Yorkshire accent (which in no way measured up to his visual image): 'Have to' play cricket.'

That leaves me feeling *very* bloody wanted. Why not just say: 'I can't be arsed'?

He insisted that we e-mail each other and he sent some very fetching fashion shoot photos while I told him to access my website and peruse the size of the job he had to tackle. Ah the luxury of it all! (Wish I had that facility: mind you, were attractiveness to be my criteria of would-be patrons I'd bloody starve to death.)

The content of his next e-mail encapsulated to me all that is wrong with the 'gun for hire' industry.

'Saw your website but couldn't see any of you wearing strappy high heeled shoes,' he whined. 'I *like* strappy shoes.'

My response was along the lines of 'Since I'm the paying customer it doesn't matter if I wear callipers and orthopaedic shoes.' (I have never mastered the art of mincing my words).

Four lotto draws later, Mr F surfaces with profuse apologies re: 'lack of communication; mix up at the office; mobile having been stolen; replacement phone in bad service area; car having tyres refitted' and all those hilarious excuses from the 'lexicon of lies' that men dip into from time to time.

Three minutes before prearranged time of appointment he rang with the most used lexicon lie of being stuck in traffic and he was at least *one and a half hours* away. In man hours that's two and a half.

I aborted the mission, reasoning that by the time he did manage to extricate himself from the M25 ring road I would be onto my second bottle of fizz and would therefore have great difficulty achieving an orgasm.

It was becoming most clear, that to these (admittedly) handsome men the escorting of women was a mere hobby (like stamp collecting) or a flight of fancy to fuck new women (when *they* felt like it) and get paid for the privilege. This is not what I want at all. The focus must be on *me, me,me*.

Another week passes. Time marches on (all over my face) Winter is slowly changing to spring (when a young man's fancy turns to *lurve*) – tides are ebbing and flowing with the waxing and waning of the moon with no reasonable expectation of getting laid by the time I attain my pensioner bus pass. Boy this is tough! Tumbleweed metaphorically rolls through my unattended vagina and my clitoris (were it to be a human being) dolefully gazes at its watch and stamps its foot with impatience. Were the situation to be reversed, would-be male customers would be bitterly complaining to OFPRO (an imaginary sex worker's ombudsman) about the time it takes to find a willing participant.

Bratislava turns to Slovenia, Milan turns to Paris and my libido throws a wobbly. Talk about 'couldn't get laid in a brothel', I can't even *pay* for it. Equality – pig's arse! I decide to put the idea to bed for a while (well at least an *idea* is being bedded) but find that I'm becoming increasingly incensed as the days pass. A juicy T-bone is tantalisingly whetting my appetite, but the quantum leap from kitchen to my plate seems impossible. Not clever and not funny: my Wendy house is not amused. Time and pussy wait for no man.

Ten days later Lena calls to say that C is back from his modelling shoot and will ring shortly Hurrah! God is good; God is great and ever so merciful. Thank you Jesus.

'Well,' I think to myself, 'I'm on the home straight now.' No retreat and no surrender. I buff and puff and generally have a total body spring clean from top-to-toe in readiness for Mr C; my 'I can make you feel *real* good' lothario. In the interim he (incongruously) sends me an email of . . . well, goodness! It looked like a cock only bigger (it took *ages* to download). Letitcia, I thought, you are a dead woman. Undeterred (even by someone who obviously loves his beef bayonet) I finally meet him.

He's active and attractive, well groomed *although smelling just the wrong side of masculine for me,* and we sally forth into the night to lock eyes over exorbitantly priced nouvelle cuisine. I very swiftly ascertain that he likes oral sex (giving). That'll do for me, pal. A £150 feast has never been devoured more quickly or with (on my part) more urgency. Back to momma bear's lair and then . . . and then . . . *it's Sheridan sheet boy!*

Let me explain.

In Australia the ad-men realised that putting a good sort (or as the Aussie women would describe 'a real spunk') on the front of either a sheet/duvet/pillowcase packet would *triple their sales* due to the 'pink dollar' being both abundant and available. These models always struck the same pose. One arm behind the head showing pythonesque biceps and looking as if they were in mid-'five knuckle shuffle' (wank). And *that* was awaiting me on my mink covered bed.

One would logically assume that since I was paying the equivalent of the Nigerian national debt, the 'hired help' would deem it his responsibility, nay *duty* to perform enthusiastically and proceed to leave no sexual stone unturned. But no. Mr Sheridan was striking a pose waiting for me to suck his 'tool of oppression'

'Some busman's holiday this has turned out to be,' I thought. Therefore to grease the wheel of absent passion, I turned somewhat proactive and proceeded to do my 'sweet thang'.

Now I care not a jot if one *is* an underwear model but *back sac and crack* is a tad of a give-away. This, along with a general reluctance to snog, a fondness for doggie and the most cursory and perfunctory licking I've had in my life (and there have been many contenders for that title) I finally twigged. He was a bloody poof!

How did he think he would get away with it? Being a woman of integrity I begrudgingly handed over the agreed king's ransom, and being a coward who dislikes confrontation I didn't even mention that he was in fact leaving six hours earlier than had been negotiated. He must be one of God's complete arseholes

Concept: if you step forward to be a male escort for women the same rules of engagement apply: I pay you money, you kiss, caress, nuzzle, stroke, lick *every* inch of my body and then give me the seeing to of my life.*That's the deal.* But oh no, these narcissistic, self-absorbed and obsessed plonkers dismissively tear up that quaint little (not unfair) rulebook with gusto.

Becoming a lesbian was, albeit fleetingly, an attractive option. But I figured the requisite four stone weight gain would put me in the morbidly obese category and the permanent scowl, which seems to be the minimum requirement for the sisterhood, would cause the very wrinkles I have spent fortunes trying to allay.

Bad idea.

One month later, having bitterly complained to head honcho at the agency that 'if they're not up for the gig then the least they could do out of professional courtesy is to sodding well pretend', Mr A is back from movie making in Paris and I prepare with leaden heart to jump through more hoops of sexual disappointment. What a saddo I am!

'Mind you,' I thought, 'he's an actor, so if he finds the prospect of living up to my (not unreasonable) expectations in any way unpalatable he can knock himself out honing his craft. He can frigging well act for goodness' sake.'

D-Day looms and I find myself going through the same two hours in the bathroom routine and I dolefully think, 'I hope he's doing this for *me*.' The prospect of a second date disaster occurring makes me practically break out in hives.

I need not have worried. He bounded up my staircase like an enthusiastic labrador. This was pay dirt with balls – sex on a very tall and turgid stick. The man was a GOD.

'If he has a brain,' I thought, there is no justice in the world.' We have ignition, lift off and, gosh oh golly, that tower has finally been cleared – whatta ride, whatta ride. *Signing off, Houston!*

A lady never kisses and tells. Commiserations, but I refuse to furnish you with the 'ins and outs of a cat's bum' regarding my date with male escort destiny. (Get your own. If you can).

But, the man was so good-looking it made you want to weep. Embarrassment seared my consciousness: I could not look this demi god in the eye. I burned with the shame of knowing I was the equivalent of a warthog to Bambi made flesh. To lose sight of this fantastic creature whilst he gave head was a travesty. I was determined to make the adjustment. To carve a monument to this epitome of manhood would have depleted the stone supply at Mount Rushmore.

He was filth with wings, a touch so deft he would have given bomb disposal a run for their money. Alexander the Great, Adonis and David? Pah! This was sheer fantasy made real in my world for a few hundred quid. He deserved ten times more. Persistence truly is the key. Sling enough shite against the wall and some will surely stick.

The trouble is he's off again to finish filming in Prague.

This whole game of attempting to give women what they want is fraught with those that think we may be so desperate and loaded we can't tell the difference. Any woman who wants male companionship will never attain the standard that is afforded the males seeking the latter. Fact.

The expression 'If you want anything doing you have to do it your self' has never been more poignant and true. Now where's my lubricant and Rampant Rabbit? Yes, the Rolling Stones were right on the money: 'You can't always get what you want, but if you pay sometimes you get what you need.'

Six Degrees of Gravy

While slithering hither and thither over a new patron's body I whispered seductively in his ear, 'Would you like some more?'

'Yes,' he croaked, 'as long as it will not deprive your other customers.'

Thereby hangs the most convoluted tale. Sad but true in this 'we pray you don't understand the concept of good service' world.

It is traditional on a Sunday, for me to visit my local bar/restaurant. Roasts, drinks and banter with the friendly staff are de rigueur. All was well until my lunch arrived. It was *sans* the usual amount of gravy. I ordered more, and a pathetic dribble nestling in the bottom of a jug was proffered. Gamefully ploughing on through my tough and dry meal, I asked once more for respite with regard to extra moisture (which is always nice).

A gruff and surly response from my server was thus: 'You can't have any more. We haven't made enough gravy and therefore, due to the abundance of bookings we have today, were we to give you more the other people would have to do without.'

I looked at her, crestfallen, and wondered if I was in the middle of a reality TV joke when she looked down at my plate and continued with her unique offhand manner: 'Anyway, it's swimming in it.'

Well that told me didn't it? Dale Carnegie's tome had obviously passed her by – winning any friends and influencing people would have been beyond her comprehension. Talk about the tail wagging the dog.

I haven't been told how to eat my food in how much or little quantities since my mother (shades of 'mommie dearest'), sat me at the table and proclaimed that I would not leave until I had finished. (Guess who won *that* battle of wills.)

Sitting in a state of astonishment, coupled with a feeling of acute humiliation ('You greedy pig ,how dare you ask for more?') I am mortified to say that my lower, upper and every lip I have in my body trembled. I had been royally 'dissed' by a waitress with major customer relation issues.

Apologies were made. Tissues were provided. Damage done. I left the premises stating (for the first time in my life) 'I'm *not* paying.' A meeting with the manageress on a Monday turned into a pow-wow with the owner on a Tuesday (sounds like a Craig David song to me). By Wednesday the die was cast: heads would be rockin' and a rollin'. By Thursday half the staff had chucked the pram toys and skedaddled in a pathetic show of solidarity.

Concept: The customer is always right. Even if he/she is wrong.

Imagine the commotion were the following scenario to take place:

'Easy, Letitcia!.You nearly made me come and I haven't got inside you yet.'

'Sorry,' I reply, 'but I don't have enough condoms and I have other bookings this evening. If I let you use one there won't be enough to go round – I'm sure you understand.'

Now I pride myself with being charming (some would say manipulative) in a sticky situation. However, there isn't enough sugar-coated, pretty please-honey in the world to diffuse what would surly be the advent of World War Three. Lalique crystal would fly and I would be remarkably lucky not to be in traction on the emergency ward at the local hospital – not to mention the ignominy of being stripped of my three stars Michelin good suck rating.

There is the premise of *six degrees of separation*, but my, that degree was so acute at my favoured Sunday lunch local it was an incestuous fraction. How was I to know the inter-personal relations of at least four of the protagonists? As in boyfriend/girlfriend, girlfriend/girlfriend and, for all I know, swapsies whenever the mood takes over. You just never know whom you are engaging with on this planet.

The saying goes: 'There is no such thing as strangers – only friends you have yet to meet.' There should be an addendum that: 'There's no such thing as well and truly not putting your foot in it, if you are not familiar with how the land lies.'

To illustrate this point perfectly let me drag you back to that den of moneymaking in Surrey Hills, Sydney. Sitting in the girls' room, we were talking (strangely) about cocks. Most of the ladies left to go and 'strut their sweet stuff' and I innocently carried on the conversation with Heidi from Germany.

'You should have been here a couple of weeks ago' I enthused. 'This guy had the biggest cock I have ever seen.'

'Damn,' she replied, 'I was on holiday.'

'Well, keep an eye out for him, gal. It's a baby's-arm-holding-an-apple type dick – and the best thing about it is, he's black.'

'Ooohhh,' she squealed, 'I just love chocolate – my boyfriend's coloured.'

'Really?' I replied. 'Well this one is very well spoken. He was born in Namibia and now earns his living selling Italian shoes all over the world . . .'

Heidi's face went white and she ran to the nearest available toilet to throw up. Clever me!

Mr Long Shlong Silver was in fact her erstwhile lover, and while she had visited relatives in her homeland he had got jiggywithit at her place of employment with *moi* truly. What a drongo! Who knew?

In fact I even adopted my present working name due to the six-degree method. Returning from Australia with nothing but memories, shared experiences, heartache and zilch in the bank, I applied for a job in the local massage parlour. *How the mighty had fallen.*

The voice that greeted me on the other end of the phone was that of a lover (lesbian) of my former supervisor (lesbian, I assume) in Oz. This lady's name was Letitcia. Since being offered the job meant I could not use my real name (another girl was already using it as her moniker) I adopted the above. This is truly a global set of fortunate circumstances. Lucky she wasn't named Ermintrude.

Reel back twenty years to England, and I'm the toast of the town, fashion-wise. Innovative, cutting edge, no one else had the balls to try and sell it – *it* being flamboyant clothes, which one would need an overpaid bodyguard to protect from the ignorant and closed minded: what *does* she look like?

Very often husbands would patronise my boutique and pick out something for 'the little lady' and, in passing, pick out something for themselves. Namely *me*. I was naive and foolish and stupidly thought it was good for business (twit). One of the husbands invited me to a gathering at his terribly trendy loft-style apartment, which in those days was the height of sophistication.

The wine flowed and so did a torrent of idiocy from my lips, directed at anyone who cared to listen. I started bragging to this attractive lady about the shoes and clothes, which the host had bought for me on a clandestine trip to BIBA. (Now that was many moons ago.)

Even though I was undoubtedly 'merry' I did have the nous to ascertain who the little lady of the house was – and fortunately it wasn't her. *Unfortunately* it was his mistress. An incident of gargantuan proportions began in earnest. I consumed my own body weight in more alcoholic beverages, and judging from the shouting and sobbing from the bedrooms so did the cuckolded female lover.

The wife finally decided to find out what the commotion was about. I passed out in a 'blue nun' haze, and the jig was up. Lover spills beans to missus, she (the missus) searches for me to corroborate story and as I come round I can hear the words the wife uttered to this day: 'Take her home, Robert, and don't bother coming back. This is not your home any longer.'

Way to go Letitcia, I hear you say – three partnerships of varying degrees destroyed in one fell swoop. Say what you will about me but I'm very time efficient. Actually the number of casualties rose to four, to include my business. Word got round that I was shagging all my customer's husbands (true, but they started it) and the well-heeled ladies that lunched, voted with their wallet and abandoned my shop in droves. Not only can I talk the hind legs off a donkey, I can kill the beast.

But stuff them if they couldn't take a joke: how the hell was I supposed to *know* all this?

Even a former boyfriend fell by the wayside of the six degrees rule. He was a womanising-gambling-lying-cheating-conniving son of a Chinaman – no, he really *was* Chinese. (I hasten to add that with maturity I have been economical with the selection process of men – I simply don't bother.)

This is how it was. He'd been schtooping, unbeknownst to me, some tart in a casino that he frequented. Well, you guessed it: her sister was a working lady in a rival brothel. He visited said brothel and found that he couldn't get laid in it (sisters do talk). He came to visit me and I wasn't coming across with the goods either!

There's a fellowship among working girls of sorts, and one phone call from sis to poor unsuspecting yours truly meant that he was forced to take his prolific philandering elsewhere.

We may as well roam the universe like traumatised mutes and take a vow of silence (becoming a Carmelite nun is becoming most appealing). Silence, like a shower, is golden.

If loose lips sink ships, I could sink an Armada . . .

Turgid Conscience

My band of co-workers crowed: 'Told you he'd be back!' He had unquestionably the face of the most gorgeous angel on this planet and that angel looked like the delectable and delovely Keanu Reeves.

He also had cerebral palsy and was wheelchair bound.

As mentioned earlier, it was customary from time to time for the specially fitted mini-van of the Valcluse home for disabled (and their carers) to visit our establishment for a jolly. It was without doubt one of the most rewarding (spiritually) and humbling experiences one will ever encounter on this mortal coil.

At first I did not feel equipped to deal with the enormity of the situation. To show affection and compassion for a grotesque was not something I had been asked to do before. Erring on the side of 'I will be a complete wuss if I do not give it a try' I attempted to reach out and touch somebody's shaking hand.

The beautiful boy chose me (though his disability was so severe he couldn't actually point). Now these unfortunate guys wanted to do the same as an able-bodied person. And it was quite a feat to accommodate a contorted writhing body (them, not me). Sometimes it was easier for the production number to be carried out while they were still in the wheel chair, which really does concentrate one's balancing powers.

I was half way through providing succour to Keanu's 'doppelganger', when a situation occurred which might have had far reaching consequences. While he busied himself nuzzling my alabaster orbs, a sharp knock was heard on the door. The involuntary response was for him to bite down in fright upon my schoolgirl type pink and perfect nipples. I in turn screamed, which set up a never-ending train of events: *bite-scream, bite-sceam, bite-scream. . .*

A bull terrier would not have had the same tenacity! I don't know what stopped this chow-down melt-down (either he ran out of bite or I ran out of tit), but order was finally restored. Apologies from carers, palsy boy with a suck under his disabled belt . . . job done. I felt good about myself. 'Who else,' I thought 'would take the time to care, and endanger one's left nipple in the process?'

So here he was once again. I rubbed some Xylocaine on my mammaries just in case, and prepared to be a sexual Mother Teresa once more. 'Hell,' I thought, 'I might even go to heaven for this unselfish act alone.'

I need not have congratulated myself so soon. He picked someone else. 'Fuck me,' I concluded, 'he's blind as well'. And there you have it. I will always cite this case, to my dying day, as an example of how men and their dicks have no rhyme or reason. I had been 'loving angel of mercy' personified and *I had been rejected by a cripple.* That just about says it all.

No sense of gratitude. No feelings of loyalty. No fidelity.

'Well, he can lick my left one,' I mentally fumed. I refused to see him again (tarts have hearts and feelings, too). Like, he has ssssoooo many mother loving options.

Sexual loyalty from a man: now *there's* an oxymoron.

When my mother was 'courting' my father, she got wind of the fact that he was actually stepping out with a few more young country ladies. She announced with hurt tones: 'I'm not going to play second fiddle.'

My charming verbose dad replied: 'Sure, you're lucky to be in the band at all!'

Then I'm sure he knuckled under the tyranny of married life (nobody can conceive the fact that their parents may have been unfaithful to one another). Take the case of those lovely little furry critters, the prairie voles. They meet, they mate for an uninterrupted 36–48 hr session and then they emit an involuntary secretion which welds them to one another for life. Ahhh, isn't nature wonderful?

In Australia Dr Glen, a Ferrari-driving gynaecologist (I hasten to add that he practised in a surgery) was a perfect example. Young, good-looking (his personalised number plate was WASTED) he had a new pretty wife, twins and another baby on the way. The man nailed every woman on the eastern seaboard of Australia. He validated his sexual wantonness in this way: 'If it's in another state it doesn't count.' Well that's all right then.

The same twisted logic comes into play in the movie-making industry: 'If it's on location it also doesn't count.' The self-delusion is quite astounding.

A punter was just about to leave (after a supreme knob polishing) when I enquired what he would be doing for the rest of the evening. He replied: 'The girlfriend will have my tea on the table by the time I get home.' Seeing my bemused look, he continued: 'Oh, don't get me wrong, I don't consider what we just did as being unfaithful.' Fanbloodytastic. I'm sure the little lady of the house will feel okay that it was only my lips rather that my labia round her man's cock.

The late James Goldsmith was quoted as saying that when you marry your mistress you immediately create a job opening. Entire societies around the world thrive on the notion that the man can (make that *will*) have what ever he wants 'on the side' as a patriarchal-given right. (As for the Muslim issue, don't get me started. Maybe in another chapter, when I can write with fury until my fingers bleed.)

In Japan the ladies are (or were) resigned to being the wife and accommodating the very thought of a mistress and some of 'mama-san's' finest at the local hostelry of professional hostesses. My God, the Ginza in Tokyo is practically a *city* devoted to male ego or cock (whichever is bigger).

I experienced the inequality my self on a foray to Nipponland. On arrival at Narita airport I pulled male company within minutes of clearing customs. (I was a speedy worker in those days.) Tetsuya Maranoushi was his name and he (being a session musician for Earth ,Wind and Fire) had flown in from LA to visit his parents in the sprawling 'burbs' of the metropolis that is Kyoto. Coffee at the airport was followed the next day by a shopping and sightseeing tour followed by (naturally) a touch of futon fumbling.

Ten out of ten for not only providing his own condom but making me come at least three times before he deemed it *his* turn for the ultimate pleasure (more of which in another chapter).

The next morning at reception I was presented with an extortionate bill for the temerity of exercising *my* right to licky-lucky oriental hospitality. I mean how *dare* I have fun with a man in my micro-sized room? The hotel staff's expressions were a picture. Frowning is not the word – a barely concealed look of distain reigned supreme. I had unwittingly broken the taboo of 'Thou shalt kneel in supplication at the feet of a man who is used to having what he wants'. Instead (how silly of me) I had deemed *my* pleasure as being of paramount importance – that showed me, didn't it?

In France the 'other woman' rocks up at births, deaths and marriage ceremonies without so much as a catfight with the Number one wife. (Shame: that would be quite a spectacle.).You cannot, however have a bit on the side unless you have installed a permanent female fixture.

That same woman is *totally complicit* in standing for the bloody nonsense in the first place.

A regular customer asserted to me the other day: 'Without my wife I'd be nothing.'

'So you mean you could derive little pleasure from your extra-curricular shenanigans if you didn't know she was biding her time in your mock-Tudor, lead-lighted, rich man's abode waiting for you to come home?'

'Precisely,' he beamed.

With a look of bemusement writ large across my face I said, 'So because you have a loving wife, you feel confident enough to see other women?'

'And if she left me I wouldn't be coming to see you.'

'You are truly a disturbed human being,' I replied.

Going for the jugular I (not so innocently) asked: 'And if she did the same, that would obviously be okay with you?'

'Don't be ridiculous,' he snorted, 'she would be thrown out of the house and I would make damn sure I got the kids.' He then (rather patronisingly I thought) added the killer line: 'Look, I don't expect you to understand this. It's *what men do*, all right?'

Aaaah, thank you for pointing that out. *Now* I understand! (Facetious, moi?) There's a standard explanation (excuse) trotted out with monotonous regularity that man is programmed to spread his seed far and wide for the purpose of procreation. Then *how do you explain blow-jobs, smarty pants?* Must be an oral immaculate conception.

Men it seems can end up with 'sweet poontang' without even wanting or consciously searching for it. I met an adorable man only the other month. A racehorse owner, he was scanning the racing pages on the internet. One of those pesky pop-ups appeared and showed a London sex site. I was affiliated to the Brighton arm and, Bob's your main man, he arrived a mere 30 minutes later – from horse to whore in three clicks.

In conclusion of this brief discourse on men's God-given right to spread their seed (and misery) at will, I will take you to an evening with a young man who I would describe as one of 'my designated fucks'. (A 'DF' is a customer with whom I like to spend more time than is financially possible on their part, and therefore I throw the occasional 'mercy fuck' their way when it suits me.)

He has a 'significant other' and the last time he came a-calling he was horrendously late to meet her in a pub. Consequently he called me in a 'post-domestic row act of contrition' to say he would have to be 'a good boy' (yeah, right) for the foreseeable future (yeah, right again). Naturally, as sure as eggs are eggs, he rocked up for more frivolity and, guess what – yes, he was damn well late again!

As he scrambled around for his hastily discarded attire (while presumably dragging up a believable excuse for what would be another gross example of tardiness) I enquired: 'If you practically split up the last time your urges took over, why in God's name would you jeopardise that relationship again?'

The reply was: 'I'm just evil'.

I couldn't have put it better myself.

Revving It Up

I was brought up to be a Catholic. My father, bless him, gamefully did his best to instil in us the basic tenets of the faith with pointless cycle rides to the nearest church. For my part I just sat looking at the back of the pew wondering when all of the stupid 'Dominus forbiscums' would finish and when I could go snogging my favourite boyfriend down in the country woods.

I endured being taught the catechism, confirmation and – the acid test – being able to perform (praying wise) after dinner at my Irish uncle's home. My relatives used to drop onto their knees after the boiled bacon and cabbage to recite some arcane mantra that totally bewildered me. How gut-wrenchingly embarrassing for poor dad. He was not as devout as the Irish contingent and therefore our religious education, or lack thereof, revealed on these squirm-making occasions more holes than a power shower nozzle.

I was not remotely interested and I did not believe, especially when some pervert dressed in the 'cloak of respectability' (i.e. cassock and dog-collar) was a little, shall we say, 'familiar'.

To speak out about the Catholic Church is tantamount to blasphemy. How many lives have been blighted and damaged in the name of silence. For myself, as I got older, I just increasingly enjoyed all the unfolding scandals from around the world, documented in the newspapers, while thinking: 'Plenty good enough for you. What you sow you reap (a tract of land the size of Patagonia), you bastards.'

All of this 'You're doing it for Jesus' malarkey, or: 'Shhh! – good girl/boy, it will be our little secret (and anyhow no one will believe you)' and then 'I have sinned my Lord', as only a true penitent can sob, just cracked me up. The chickens had finally come home to roost, but I was the one crowing.

Whenever I go to visit my family, the taxi driver (and, lest we not forget, they are the ultimate font of knowledge) regales me with stories of my religious tormentor. He (the venerable frocked man) has clambered out of more windows in the event of a husband's/boyfriend's early arrival home, than the swagman himself.

I suppose the problem lies in the premise of 'we are above the common urges of carnality. If you have made a vow of celibacy then you've surely made not a monkey, but a raving great gorilla for your back.

Those that can, fuck – and those that cannot, proceed to pontificate and moralise in the ultimate hypocritical way. How do they keep a straight face?

'Bless me father, for I have sinned.'

'And how long is it since your last confession?'

'Oh, well – shall we say 30 years?'

'Well jump on my lap and we'll talk about it my child.'

How fabulous to be able to wipe away all of one's indiscretions with a bit of Hows-yer-father and Hailing-yer-Mary: a very cunning stunt. Whoever makes up these rules of engagement (and they must truly be made up on the spot, in a blind panic) must be laughing all the way to a wank.

Here follows a true story (documented in a red-top tabloid), which illustrates the arrogance of some of the papal people.

I used to have my follicles fiddled with (that's hairdressing to you) by a very camp young man called Mark. His boyfriend was a vicar. I can't remember which branch of the religious tree forbids sex with a woman or indeed the 'love that dare not scream its name'. Whatever, they were surely doing it.

'What do they say,' I enquired, 'when you check into a hotel together?'

Mr arrogant vicar replied smugly 'No one questions a dog collar.'

(Perhaps all the villains in the world could employ that small tactic. As squad cars screech to the scene of some heinous crime, they would almost certainly back away when confronted with this vital piece of gravitas-giving apparel. Were it to be *that* simple you could get away with what many religious dick-heads have been for centuries – robbing money and fiddling with sons and daughters. And as for the Sisters of Mercy, make that Nazis in drag. But I digress.)

I rented a flat from the terrible toxic twins for the purposes of isolating my private life from my privates. It went not pear-shaped but the most bloody great cantaloupe you have ever imagined. Blue rinsed dowagers were appalled (no, make that *aghast*) that I in my leather lace and chains had somehow crumpled their neighbourhood's seamless financially cushioned existence.

A disgruntled ex-employer (lesbian) took a dim view of an employee (me) going solo. (I think you might just find that is termed in the statute books as 'controlling'.) Some benevolent soul took it upon him/herself to inform the national press of a scandal unfolding. (The combination of vicar/tart is irresistible.)

Oh, and I forgot to mention, unbeknown to me my father was in hospital dying of prostate cancer.

Hurrah, bring it on and do your worst!

Reporters tracked down Mr Holier-than-thou and Nancy-boy crimper and the jig was up. I disbanded my 'business', went to spend the next few days on a deathbed vigil and the newspapers came up with the headline:

KINKY TART SELLS BODY WORSHIP AT VICAR'S POSH FLAT.

Oh joy, oh rapture. After dad's burial I returned to find all the taxi drivers in Brighton leering and leching into their rear-view mirror, pronouncing proudly 'Saw you in the newspaper the other day.'

'Yes,' I thought 'must be some achievement to read the *Sun* whilst munching a hamburger. You really should be awarded a medal proclaiming you to be *champion dolt.*'

Since I wasn't 'working' I thought it might be a good idea to collect the remaining eight weeks' rent that I had given to the greedy duo. Fat chance! Phone calls were avoided and the penultimate conversation with the mink-wearing, priest-sucking nancy boy was 'He feels you've brought it all on yourself and therefore we don't feel obliged to repay your advance rent.'

No compassion there, then.

There's an intriguing postscript to this tale of Tally'ho. The rev was struck off/ousted by his own church for, shall we say, misappropriating vulnerable parishioners' possessions. With unerring regularity the dying (he being chaplain at a local hospital) were mysteriously signing over their worldly goods to this dreadful man and his accomplice. The police, because of complaints from distressed relatives, have still not proved the case. But give it time baby, because greed and avarice never sleep. And when that day arrives (and it will) 'twill be a case of *Bless me father, for I have grinned.*

Drop the AK 47 (Disarm today, Datarm tomorrow)

A few days ago, after a good nights sleep, I switched on my mobile phone to see what the new day would bring. My voicemail had recorded this message: *'Fucking bitch.'* One hour later, while sauntering to the shops, another voice shouted in my ear *'Fucking bitch'* – and it was barely 9.30 am. As starts to the day go, it wasn't one of my best. (A wank and three cuppas do it for me, though the latter will suffice if under time constraints.)

The second voice was from a bitter twisted homosexual (I obviously represent to him the spawn of the devil.) The first (female) voice was from the wife/girlfriend of a patron. He had omitted to inform her that he was 'playing away from home' and she, being suspicious, went through his mobile phone for recently called numbers and texts. When interrogated by 'outraged of Burgess Hill' I lapsed immediately into that standard flanking deployment of *deny, deny, deny*. After all, it seems to work for men!

What occurred to me was the amount of hate and misdirected animosity there is in this world. Freedom fighters, faces contorted with naked vitriol and blood lust – these guys sssooo need a good seeing to,' I muse.

Apparently it takes more muscles to frown than to smile, so all those miserable buggers out there could end up (botox notwithstanding) looking like the most lugubrious boxer dog on this unsettled planet. Whenever I see news clips of whichever country is currently tearing itself apart I always whimsically think that what all these invective-filled young men need is a good suck.

An Italian porn star (La Ciccolina), actually offered her professional services (in the name of humanity) to 'old happy bollocks', Mr Saddam Hussein, when the advent of the first Gulf war was looming. My goodness – to coin a phrase from that most wonderful of movies, Casablanca – 'in her own way she could have constituted an entire second front'. It might have shaped history.

'Excuse me your excellent and most wonderful ruler: we need the order to strike.'

Saddam, watching the blonde temptress's anus gliding up and down on his camel-sized cock, would probably have replied: 'Nah, let's call the whole thing off. Can't you see I'm on a roll here? I'm in an ecstatic state of Don't bug me.'

Mind you, consummate professional as I am, I would have baulked at having to administer pleasure to Saddam's favourite son Uday. Rumour has it that that if the designated totty was not up to his high or insane standards, then it was 'goodnight Vienna'. (A blow-job can be problematic enough re teeth displacement and gag reaction.) The prospect of being beheaded, were the experience deemed not up to scratch wouldn't elicit my best sexual performance. I felt sorry for the footballers in the Iraqi national football team. – fancy playing with wobbly legs and soiled underwear.

Orgasms are the opiate of the masses. Well, that's what I think. Many have been the days when I have been incapable of walking or even talking, so high am I on the release of a 'sex drug'. God bless you climax givers wherever you are (princes among men, every one of you).

Since men generally visit working women to relax and forget about their woes, it follows that governments currently engaging in wholesale slaughter around the world should be sent B-52s absolutely filled with hookers (or amateurs with a social/political conscience). Forget the extra personnel and sons and daughters coming home in body bags. Getting laid is where it's at. Lets blitz the war zones with clits. Fill the battlefield with babes.

'Corporal, secure that ridge immediately!'

'Sorry Sarge, can't be arsed. That little minx sucked me dry and I'm feeling rather fluffy. Fact is, I feel nothing but goodwill toward men.'

It's that simple.

When you climax the brain sends a message to the pituitary gland and that wonderful secretion, endorphin (the body's natural morphine) gives you a Weetabix glow. (My mate Harry informs me that it's a Ready Brek glow but I speak as I find, and that's the stuff I was bought up on.)

I have never succumbed to the taking of heroin, but I have heard accounts from ex-users and read testimonials from trustworthy or, should I say noteworthy, journalists. I am told one feels sheer bliss, or that it's like being wrapped in cotton wool. Well, that's how I feel when I come. (Don't tell me I am the exception to the rule.)

The Japanese had their comfort women. The Germans had the Jews, the Poles and any poor sod who happened to be incarcerated. The Americans had (by all accounts) half the English women under the age of ninety. They were 'over-sexed and over here', and, enterprisingly, they could lay their hands on a pair of silk stockings and (if they really liked you) a packet of Lucky Strike ciggies. Though it didn't actually stop them from engaging in battle, at least they killed with a smile on their face, a song in their heart and probably a nasty rash on their bell end. As for the British, I'm sure the only stiff thing was the upper lip. Well, we wouldn't go in for the 'horizontal mambo' would we? Heaven forefend: we are made of sterner stuff. (Think Alec Guinness in 'Bridge Over the River Kwai'.)

My father opined that the state of the world was, in part, the result of two major world wars. Train a man to be a lean, mean killing machine and how does he stop? Well now they need commando training in the 'karma sutra'. De-programme the monsters we have created. Brainwash them, (those unfortunates who ultimately do the master's bidding and pay dearly for it) with the 'make love not war' ideology.

Both practical and oral. (I'll take the oral.) If we reprogrammed the pugilistic armies to make lovarama instead of that tedious 'machinegun-machete one/two', the Arab women would not be wailing for their fallen relatives but merely for the shame and ignominy of the pregnant ladies in their midst.

Make love, not war. Nobody ever died from making love. (Except, I know the autoeroticists and those with a dodgy ticker who have fallen foul). But when the skies are lit with rocket fire, bomb shrapnel is exploding and bullets are ricocheting you know what the deal is. With a bit of slap and tickle the worst that can befall you is a trip to the local clap clinic, the morning after pill or (worse) a marriage proposal.

I cannot believe that an enterprising politician has not thought of it before. The exploits of sirens, *femmes fatales* and honey trappers have been well documented. Now's the time to execute a bold plan. Come on ladies – *your country needs you*. You know you love a man in uniform.

Men make the quarrels but it's the women and children that bear them, so rage against the patriarchal machine. Remember (and this is a personal motto) that 'you catch more flies with honey than with than with pig shite'. A woman with an amorous agenda is both a terrifying and formidable force. Hell, it's not even a fair contest. If a man will have sex and hang the consequences waiting at home (re the wife standing with an irate expression and a baseball bat in her hand), then the sergeant majors and generals will be a piece of piss.

There *is* an alternative, but none as pleasurable.

Talking to one of my beauticians I learned that, sadly, it was her last day due to the fact that her father was dying with bone cancer, which was the progression of a prostate condition. Since my own father had been afflicted with the same disease, I asked whether his mood changed with the anti-cancer drugs routinely prescribed. She said they had, and he was a much softer, nicer, more approachable person. He had been injected with the female hormone oestrogen – into his testicles. (Prostate cancer apparently feeds and grows on the male hormone, testosterone.)

Ladies, which would you prefer – administering a prick or receiving one? Yes, right, I thought so.

Action, not words. Good old Kofi could retire and Blair's 'third way' would be no way at all.

A Smith & Wesson beats four aces and a disillusioned cock will 'run home to momma'. You have to endure intensive training to be a warrior, but to rut and fornicate is instinctive – so we have the edge.

For bad things to prosper all that is required is for good men/women to do nothing – and the prospect of a heaving, passionate coming together (especially in wartime) must surely be too much to resist.

Long live Punani Power!

Slap My Thigh and Ride in on the Wave

'**M**en love big women, and want them in the bedroom for sure, but they don't want to be seen with a fat tart by their mates,' opined Leslie.

'Well, I think I'm anorexic,' said Christina with a wicked smile.

'And how do you figure that one?' I spluttered (for she must be 14 stone).

'Every time I look in the mirror all I see is a fat person.'

How we laughed!

This being just one subject up for ridicule and discussion.

Sunday, and another lunch where taboo subjects are given an airing. My mate, 'the lesbian fluffer from hell' Christina, Leslie and I preside over a table groaning with fine wines/champagnes and, for me, *cranberry juice*. Well, they don't call cystitis the honeymoon syndrome for nothing, and it had been a heavy week.

'I think a large lady who is comfortable with her weight is infinitely more attractive to men than a skinny-Minnie, who looks like the 3.15 entry at the Haringey [greyhound] race track,' I reasoned. 'Besides, I'm not overweight, just under *height*.'

'I purposely put on weight to stop being attractive to men,' Christina countered.

'Did it work?' I asked.

'Well, I'm now a lesbian,' she chuckled.

A few weeks ago I was languishing in the arms of a handsome young man (*another shitty day in paradise*) who decided that Saturday night on the town was no longer cutting the mustard. He was mightily tired of spending half his disposable income standing in bars that he didn't like, drinking alcohol that he didn't want and ingesting smoke fumes which his body couldn't stand. All in the name of getting laid.

He did the sensible thing and spent his hard earned with me. Now, entwined in post coital/orgasmic bliss, he congratulated himself on not only finding a lady who could competently deep throat, but one who was very large and voluptuous.

'I don't understand why any man bothers to try to select who is going to be the lucky winner of his affections,' I said.

'How do you mean?' he quizzed.

'Because they all look the same – same haircut, same clothes and same weight. Not one is above seven stone wringing wet.'

'Yeah, well that's the only thing that's out there at the moment. I really can't stand skinny women, and neither can my mates, but what can you do?'

He expelled a deep sigh of dissatisfaction and continued: 'They think we like them slim and we can't seem to convince them otherwise – so we end up going with birds we don't really find attractive, and they kind of pick up on the vibes and before you know it we're arguing about weight. If you want to get laid, you either have to keep your mouth shut or yer wallet open.'

And there you have it. Out of the mouths of babes.

A word in your shell-like. Watch a woman when she eats. If she's got grease/cream/gravy dripping down her chin and eats her butter-drenched (or drizzled) asparagus with sensual aplomb, then chances are *you're certain to have the time of your natural-born in the cot.* (Knowing my great love of food, my local has named a dish in my honour. It's called 'Yum yum pig's bum nut roast'. I am not making this up.) It may cost you more when you take her out for the routine 'meal before expected sex' on a Friday or Saturday night (she'll have all three courses). But boy will you have plenty of wanking material to lust over for the coming weeks: insatiable eater, insatiable lover – easy peasy, let me teasy. Oh, *do* keep up (007): do I have to teach you everything?

I once worked in the antipodes with a beautiful American girl. She probably weighed fifteen stones. Her hair was all Nicole Kidman tendrils of bleach-tipped California curls. She decided to embark on a radical change of image. She laboured each morning with a Jane Fonda workout and had her hair bleached flaxen-white & shorn a-la-Prisoner Cellblock H.

She most certainly achieved her objective, but as her weight dropped so did the number of patrons who would normally come to visit.

All of that deprivation *for nought.* She tortured herself because she thought she'd be more popular with the paying customers.

'Never underestimate the general public's taste', I believe some movie mogul once said.

Years ago (when I was young, dumb and full of everyone's cum), I too thought that slim was in. I don't know whether I was endomorph, ectomorph or mesomorph, but I was swayed by the constant images in magazines and hadn't yet developed my grown up 'id'. I very stupidly took diuretics.

Whenever I went out I literally *passed* out. Because of the lack of water in my body. I was a size ten, but I didn't have the energy to go the distance with any interested male party. Fuck that shit – that's what I think. I allow my body to do what it wants to do, and so it meanders like the tributary of the Nile, a free spirit – *free at last, free at last!*

'You don't sweat much for a fat lass'.

No, nobody has had the temerity to say it to my face, (well not if they want a blow-job anyway), but I have had the odd 'you're a big girl' from eight stone weaklings – who incidentally (from my extensive experience) have a cock that accounts for half their body weight. Being meaty can also hold untold advantages. As a young girl, the ganger and myself could always see my mother among a strawberry field-full of upturned posteriors – hers was the biggest.

Let your body do what it wants to do and a dick will follow. Stuff them if they can't take a joke. If they think they can pull supermodels, let them do their worst: I can always get a man in bed. Mind you, the date-rape drug Rohypnol and chloroform is often called upon in dire straits (joking).

My neighbour Linda is a very petite and beautifully formed lady. Yet she confessed that when it came time to get up and go to the loo (when there was a lover lying awake in her bed) she somehow had to wrap a sheet round herself or even hold a pillow over her bum lest he saw her body.

'But, you dopey sod, you will have been doing everything known to man with one another, you'll get naked and he'll climb inside for the ride, do it in every position! You think he hasn't *seen* it already?' I argued

'I know, but I'm just not confident enough'

'Linda, petal, you're confident enough to stick your arse up in the air and have their dicks rammed so far up it practically knocks your teeth out. You don't put a pillow over your bum when you shag do you?' I asked in exasperation

'No, I just bite it when it hits the cervix' she replied sarcastically.

'I know,' I enthused. 'Crawl on all fours to the loo – that way he'll see exactly the view he's been mounting.'

'Now you're being silly.'

'I'm not the one wearing a yashmak to the toilet.'

There are certain countries around the world, where the larger, curvier female is the most revered of the species. (I can hear the ladies shouting: 'Book me a ticket right now'). Yet, though I have travelled extensively, I have never felt the need to go to these havens of bigger women. I have never felt that had I been smaller, or more gym-honed, that I would have attained the attention of the man I wanted to sleep with. Pah! When all else fails I *laugh* them into bed (as my mate Harry does).

There is no bigger compliment than being paid by beautiful young men to make love. (It's a filthy job, but . . .). They're not isolated incidents and nor are they one-offs. I often muse that they return again to see if it really *was* that bad the first time round! Even though I know I have been the subject of a 'bet' by young guys (the youth of today, eh?), it hasn't been like the 'grab a granny' or 'pull a fat chick' nights that male wags embark on from time to time (or so I am assured).

Tracy, (my mate Harry's bird) is pregnant and her body shape is changing .He cannot wait to get home to schtoop her. He has never found her more attractive – she's now an object of fecundity. He is not only congratulating himself on impregnating her (he calls himself 'super sperm'), but on being able to make his dreams of a ripe curvy lover come true.

Myself, I have been medium, large and impossible. I like the fact that when I lie in bed my breasts fall into my mouth like proffered grapes – well, only a slight exaggeration. I like to envelop my lovers with soft yielding flesh. After all, 'vive la différence'. If you like spare ribs and 'lucky legs' (lucky they don't break), seek life elsewhere.

So best strap yourself in: this is going to be a bumpy night, but don't worry about any bruises.

I'm built for comfort, not for speed.

Don't Panic, Mr Mainwaring!

When the going gets weird, the weird turn pro. We all have days when things do not go according to plan. 'Tis merely the universe testing us. If we come through with flying colours, then well done us. What follows are a few examples of not 'oh dear!' but a gigantic *fucking hell, what have I done?'*

There used to be a dear, gentle soul called Chris who owned a leather workshop emporium. He revelled in making various instruments of torture and/or sexy leather apparel. Indeed, he was so heavily into pain that he used to do a tour of dentists on the pretext of having something wrong with his molars or upper bicuspids (there never *was* anything wrong). He loved the pain of well-meaning dentists drilling into his nerves (ouch!), and figured that for £37.50, which was the going national health rate, it was cheaper than going to see a professional dominatrix.

He loved nothing more than making up inventions of pain or restraint for the sex trade, and I bought one or two myself. I think fondly of him whenever I don my bespoke 'Bitch' dog-collar. Lamentably, he hanged himself.

But his creations live on. One was called 'the crucible'.

In my abode on a sunny summer's afternoon a few years ago, there stood a trembling man. He was sweating with terror. The crucible had four chains attached, on the end of each chain was a dog clip and in the centre of the crucible was 'tea light holder' – which was lit. The dog clips were pinched onto his testicles and the crucible was suspended below his dick and his gonads. The heat emanating was not enough to burn his balls (though strangely they *do* swell and drop toward heat), but it was capable of doing this to his dick if it did not stay stiff and upright. Now *that's* what you call a man under pressure.

This was a remarkably well-known man, a captain of his particular industry, as to a lesser degree was his wife – who chose that very moment to ring her betrothed dearly beloved. I challenge any homo sapien to remain hard under these trying circumstances and clearly he was struggling. If a man is trying *not* to ejaculate I normally suggest trying to think of the number of S's in Mississippi (my mate Harry thinks of cos lettuces), but I have no professional trick to make a man stay fulsome (especially in this unique circumstance).

His erection slowly dissolved with no discernable hope of the trend being reversed.

A trickle of sweat ran forlornly down the side of his cheek as he struggled to maintain his poise on the phone to his missus. His hands were bound behind his back as I held his mobile to his (sweaty) ear. With my other hand I tried to gauge how warm the flame was making his rapidly deflating dick. It was getting kind of warm down there and Mr 'Cool under any circumstance' was rapidly losing his 'savoir fair'.

'Yes dear, we'll get the plumber to sort that out next week – now I must go . . . What's that got to do with the price of fish? . . . I don't care how much it costs . . .

'Look,' he finally snapped, '*I have to go!*'

His wife obviously picked up on his edginess and cross-examined him closely. My poor customer was in abject misery. He looked pleadingly at me but I stayed in character: that of a nasty dispassionate dom.

'There's nothing wrong, why should anything be wrong' he beseeched.

Back in the danger zone things were not looking pretty, but back on the phone his wife continued her investigation – until he screamed *'Get off the phone you stupid fucking bitch!'*

On cue I disconnected the phone, but such was his agony I also tore the offending contraption from his appendages, and with it went the molten wax – all over my freshly laid mega-expensive carpet (and, I suspect, a significant part of his nether regions). His balls were singed and his todger looked worryingly as if it had first-degree burns.

Being a compassionate female, I fretted and worried about how the hell I would be able to rescue my Harrods rug from the dried wax. Meanwhile he wondered what the quickest response time for the paramedics might be whilst trying to come up with the ultimate 'lexicon lie' covering burnt genitals.

So, ladies and gentlemen, would you like to hear the lie?

'I had just stepped out of the shower to check on my grilled sausages, and since they were already well done I took the sizzling tray out while simultaneously reaching for a plate. The floor was wet and I slipped, knocking the red hot fat over my penis'. (Believe that and you'll believe anything.)

It took him a mere *three seconds* to concoct this very tall story/excuse, yet it required prompting from me to seal the preposterous lie.

'Don't forget to drop in to the butchers on the way home,' I said knowingly

'Why? Oh, bugger – of course!'

If one practises to deceive, best do it properly.

In Sydney there was a curious man called 'Germ'. He loved visiting working girls but was convinced that by merely touching us in any way (or indeed any thing we had remotely come into contact with) he would contract the most heinous disease. So he liked to watch – a hidden voyeur to the unsuspecting customer being serviced on the bed. What Germ didn't know was that a guy we called 'Germ 2' was secretly watching *him*. (A little like the modern phenomena called dogging). The working ladies thought this was a delicious secret, and there was a certain advantage to earning triple dollars due to the extra participants involved. It normally went off without a hitch, like some kind of well-oiled machine.

This sexual farce could only be carried out in one particular room, to keep up the pretence of anonymity. Germ 2 would be ensconced on the balcony (fourth floor) and concealed behind a huge antipodean shrub. Germ would be inside the French windows but behind a heavy velvet curtain, and the poor unsuspecting entertainment-provider would be treated to the time of his life just to distract him from the goings on both inside and out side the room. What jolly japes!

Then a moody knock was heard at the door. The supervisor whispered bad news: another bomb scare. When I say another, I mean thaat scares are the curse of the brothel industry. Disgruntled clients, ex-workers, boyfriends or husbands of workers, they all employed this effective tactic.

It caused mayhem. Girls wanting their night's money (lest it went up in smoke) and men wanting their money back (so they could visit a brothel where a bomb wasn't the 'blow-job du jour', or worse (for the lady) to be made to stay and finish the 'pay per screw'. As a generality these threats had to be taken seriously, though so frequent were they that 'cry wolf' had become 'cry what ever the fuck you like I'm trying to earn some dosh here'.

On this occasion, as 'Sydney's finest' raced to the scene of a potential crime, the little Aussie battler who had saved his hard-earned for his birthday (and probably divorce treat) was in for the long haul. He had paid, and I made an executive decision not to worry his pretty ugly head about the fact that not only would it be the best suck of his life, it might actually be his last, and if he had to die on the nest then gosh darn, what a way to go. I'm a pretty much a fly-by-the-seats kind of gal, though I never thought the day would come when that was literal.

Women are supposed to be super adept at multi tasking, but the King's Cross fire department and police, a punter with a mid-life crisis (or shortened life as the case may be), and two perverts who were blissfully unaware of the drama/trauma unfolding was a heavy straw on this camel's crack – first I had to deal with my birthday boy.

'Bruce,' I whispered seductively 'would you like to wear a blindfold and get into some kinky shit for your 40th birthday.'(At least he wouldn't be able to see my rising panic.)

'Strewth, you pommie women are bloody dags – sure why not? By the way, what was that knock at the door? Our time ain't over yet, is it?'

No was the metaphorical answer, but I longed to say 'We'll just have to wait and see'.

I knew that if Germ was so neurotic about disease he would have an instant heart attack if I relayed a written message to him regarding our potential imminent demise. It was strangely ironic that he thought we working girls were the harbinger of doom. Talk about the wrong place at the . . . So I hedged my bets, thinking that he had at least a 50–50 chance of it all being some elaborate hoax. This was like playing God. I also knew that if he discovered Germ 2 watching him slapping his salami, a coronary would yet again be on the cards.

So I couldn't actually dash behind the curtain and give him a note (which he wouldn't have taken due to my imagined innate pox) to relay to *his* voyeur. Oh, bums and burnt bollocks, what's a girl to do? As far as I was concerned it was every man for himself.

As for my own safety, I was in the midst of a miserable 'just split up with a man jerk' faze, and I really didn't give stuff one way or another

'Three guys having great sex while I am in my own personal hell,' I thought. Story of my life.

Then the fire brigade arrived. My blindfolded customer, hearing other voices in the room, just thought I had really pushed the boat out, in order to tantalise his senses. Germ (as I later found out) was delighted for an addition to the proceedings and upped beating his bayonet to 50 strokes a minute. And what of Germ 2? The poor man was arrested by the police as a suspected intruder in the course of their search for a bomb. The management eventually vouched for the fact that he *was* meant to be there, to withering looks from Mr Plod.

'What kind of place are you bloody running here' the constable asked me much later.

'You have *no* idea' I sighed.

A few years ago, with a different blindfold and a different man, I suffered the same cringeworthy outcome. A situation was spiralling way out of control; another disaster waited to be added to my burgeoning heap.

Poor Norman – the archetypal Mr Bean (over 40, carried shopping bag and lived at home with his mother) – had fallen foul of my 'oops' moments once before. Somehow I had mixed up his predilection for pain with somebody else's, and fitted his proud member with a very painful cock strap, with sharp teeth/ spikes on the inside. He was blindfolded at the time (some things never change) and therefore couldn't see to ask me indignantly 'What the fuck do you think you're doing?' His agonising scream was probably borne on the wind all the way to Dieppe.

I was most surprised to see him again.

Unfortunately for him, his visit coincided with the most severe attack of PMS I had ever had. I was unhinged, deranged and only just the correct side of homicidal. As far as I'm concerned the only thing more terrifying in this life is a missed period. Beneath the welcoming facade of 'Let me take your coat' or 'What refreshment would you like?' lurked a seething banshee who wanted to kill, maim, damage anything or anybody in my way.

Handcuffs were applied, the blindfold was in place and instruments of varying degrees of pain and torture,(along with a few homespun inventions of my own) were waiting to be called into service once more.

I strutted my stuff, but my mind wandered to every single negative incident that had happened in my life: every imagined slight, each nasty humiliation, all the useless sons of bitches who had brought me to my knees in tears. This maelstrom of awfulness was transferring itself to my control of the wrist action.

When a man visits a professional dominatrix there is a tacit unspoken understanding that borders will not be breached and that personal limits and tolerance will be understood. I had clearly (albeit unwittingly) lost all control.

In l[...] upon bleeding balls and a cock that was rapidl[...] e Kinte black. Don't ask how I managed to stuff u[...] arly with the same poor victim *twice*, but I surely[...] stion of how to extricate myself from this monur[...] eemed to have no suitable answers. Was he writhir[...] ecstasy? Should I charge him more for going the ext[...] ld I bribe him to keep his mouth shut? Would he go t[...]

The l[...] answered itself based on my vast reservoir of knowledge i[...] ng men, sex and the police. I can see the scene in the interview room:

'Now let me get this right, sir, you actually rang this lady of your own volition?'

'Well yes, but I didn't know that . . .'

'But sir,' the officer asks, 'you did go there to receive some sort of pain did you not?'

'Since you put it like that,' he grudgingly concedes, 'yes, I did.'

'So you had your eyes wide open.'

'No, I was blindfolded.'

The officer's question now bristles with irritation: 'Yes I know, but it seems you are merely complaining about the level of discipline. Didn't you says anything at the time, sir?'

'I had a gimp ball strapped in my mouth,' he answers.

'You stated you had visited this particular lady before – was it okay the first time?'

'No, she shoved spikes through my penis,' he complains.

'And you went back?!' he thunders. 'Jesus, you deserve every thing you get, pal – we have no case to answer here!'

Poor Mr Bean. I mopped up the ball blood and for good meassure added some germoline, which stung like a bitch. He seemed to like it. My PMS had receded to the back of my turmoil-stricken thoughts. (Funny how a drama concentrates and focuses the angst riddled mind.) I then masturbated him with ice cubes to show some belated compassion, and he seemed to like that, too. I then steeled myself for his reaction when I removed his Virgin Airways upper class blindfold.

Nothing. Nada. Zip. Nothing was mentioned. From the disgrace of a police record, a black mark on the sex offenders' register and national notoriety I rose phoenix-like from some icy ashes. He actually *loved* it. So turned on was Mr Bean by this debacle that he came to visit much more regularly.

Victory, like Viagra, is often stumbled upon accidentally . . .

Going Down Down Under

'Christ she was a real Razorback – but it was late and my balls were going blue with desire. I simply *had* to do something about it!'

My mate Fred was regaling me with stories of his recent trip to Australia and as usual the subject turned to sex.(Come to think of it, if I was forbidden to raise the subject again I would have sod all to talk about: it's my vocation and the subject matter stretches to infinity.)

'Even though I was drunk, I knew she was a bushpig,' he exclaimed, lapsing into the Aussie vernacular for 'pug ugly'.

'What happened when you got her home?' I asked.

'You don't think I'd let me mates *see* her do you?' he spat 'No, I made damn sure I went to her place, and it was in this scum-sucking, filthy hole called Redfern – d'ya know it? Ever go there?'

'I was told to avoid it at all costs,' I replied.'Isn't that where they have race riots with the indigenous people?'

'Probably. Come to think of it, she looked like an abbo.' He replied. He put his head in his hands. 'She was real triple-bagger.'

'Your command of the English language has plummeted since you went to Sydney,' I said. 'What on earth does that mean?'

'It's when a shag is so unpalatable you put one paper bag over *her* head and two over your own just in case one slips off.'

'So come on,' I pressed 'What happened?'

He looked mournful and embarrassed: 'Christ I just didn't know where to start – she'd thrown up earlier and still smelled of vomit'

'Nice,' I deadpanned. 'Sounds like a right little charmer.'

'Then I moved further down and she had more chunder in her bra!'

'You must have been desperate.'

'Wait till you hear what happened next!' he cried. 'She had this sanitary towel between her legs.'

'Oh yuck, you're grossing me out.'

'And *then* she chucked it across the bedroom and said "Sorry mate, forgot to tell ya, I'm on the blob – but I wouldn't mind youse bangin' me up the shitter" – and as I'd gone so far, I *did!*'

Welcome to sex in the Land of Oz, where the women are like men and the men are like animals. I had heard stories that I thought were apocryphal, but having spent a 10-year tenure there, I know they are absolutely true.

The ladies are bought up tough, due I imagine to the original pioneering spirit that made Aussie land what it is today.

The first time I arrived in Australia, I was so traumatised by my post-25 hour flight and stroll down William Street in Sydney, that I nearly did a volte face and skedaddled back to where the pace of life seemed more . . . well, genteel. My ears were assaulted by the monstrous sound of Strine and it was coming from the Sheilas. These women had voices that could strip paint, curdle milk and grate the hardest cheese. 'I sure would hate to wake up to *that* sound in the morning,' I thought.

The Holdens with their V.8 engines were somehow more brutal and in your face than those cars pottering around a city in old Blighty. They were Mad Max warriors, who strove to mow you down if you didn't negotiate the zebra crossing in time. Like a rabid dog they sensed my fear and reduced me to tearful, fearful wreck.

What fresh hell was this? Infected mosquito bites and unidentifiable creepy crawlies added to my misery.

So I had left Pommie-land for this. Yes, I was immediately labelled one, too, for I was moaning and whining (unfortunately not in a sexual way) day and mossie-biting night.

When the Kiwi bastard with whom I was travelling decided to visit his parents without me (what am I, chopped liver?), I did what any scorned woman would do. I got a job in Sydney's best whorehouse just to spite him.

It was there I had my introduction as to how crass the Aussie male can be in the cot. They don't have any concept of the term 'lovemaking'. They grab, grapple, prod, pull, squeeze and irritate the bejezzus out of you.

They have perfected the 'bowling ball technique' (two digits in the front and one thumb up the back) and made it their own. They also try to emulate everything they see in porn movies.

'Shit, this drongo that I had a one-hour appointment with, d'ya know what he just tried to do?' I asked.

The clutch of tarts (I believe that is the correct collective term) who congregated in the girls' room barely bothered to look up from their tabloid fodder: 'Didn't try to stick his foot up yer chuff by any chance, did he?' replied Kelly – one of the longest standing and most battle hardened hookers in the southern hemisphere. Seems 'Mr Foot' (rather than 12 inches), could not see the line between fantasy and reality, and while waiting for me he watched a racy movie where gerbils and pain and all manner of esoteric things were played out on the screen. Having watched the film in its entirety, I considered that I had got off lightly.

If a fit young male ever came through the door we would all recoil in horror at the prospect of being picked, and attempt to look as uninterested as possible. We checked our fingernails, gazed into the middle distance and stared at the floor. Every fibre of our body squealed: 'Please don't choose, me – please don't choose me.' We wouldn't look our nemesis in the eye for fear that it would be deemed an encouraging sign. 'Go away and torture someone else,' we thought.

Why?

As a generality all young guys would do the same thing once ensconced in the room. They frotted, they rooted, they shagged, pummelled, fucked and pounded with all of their brutal might. And they could do it for *hours*. It was not an act of love or even, for that matter, lust. The cervix would be relentlessly stabbed until it was reduced to pulp. We were not caressed or stroked, we were manhandled like a big hairy ewe in a sheep shearing competition. They also thought this code of conduct was de rigueur, and were one to voice a complaint of any description, they got jolly batey.

I tried to explain that 85–90 per cent of women *did not come by being fucked* – though I'm not sure if this was the reason which prompted such athleticism. This information fell on deaf ears (they were trained for this) and the poor female recipient was reduced to being an aerodynamic piece of hi-tech gym equipment. They 'worked out' like a metronome, with not so much as a by-your-leave or cursory glance in our (their) sweat-covered direction. I frankly would rather stick needles in my eyes and pull hairs out of my own anus, for that would be preferable to this endless purgatory.

One would imagine that being asked to perform oral would be a relief. But no, Aussie man plays Aussie rules in that department too. They prop up their pillows (so they can get a *real* good look at the unfortunate participant), look down with pride at their pork prodder and usually say something like: 'There you go, let's see what you can do with *that*. You'll be a while, mind – had a few tinnies before I came here.' Peachy.

And so you start. Twenty minutes into this laborious and pointless exercise and the dick-head attached to the dick would casually reach over and light up a cigarette/spliff. No embarrassment. Just the most natural thing in the world to gulp beer and inhale while a member of the opposite sex is attempting to raise the dead. Then it's a toilet break (for him) to rid him of the 15 pints previously imbibed. This brings the hard-on status back to square one. The buzzer for 'time off for good behaviour' goes and it's your entire fault they haven't expelled any 'baby batter'. They get real shitty with it and demand to see the management, who *always* rule in the customer's favour.

'Guy here says he hasn't come,' the supervisor says accusingly.

'Well it's hardly my fault he was rat arsed when he got here, he's smelly and rude and his dick is like a Chinese noodle,' I reply. 'He's never going to come.'

'He's a regular and he's spent a fair few dollars over the years. You get back in there and service him ,young lady'

You drag yourself back to your dreadfully flaccid client whose face is the picture of a triumphant sneer.

'Guess youse gotta start all over again, but before you do I gotta take a dump.'

How to give a tormentor a blow-job without yielding to the overriding urge to bite it off completely is a testament to the stoic nature of the English people. Unfortunately I'm half Irish – it was a close call on numerous occasions.

It wasn't *all* bad. There has to be a beam of light in the darkness, so step forward, you shining knights of Sydney, for I have *never* forgotten you, the 'B' division Fire Department. Yum, yum, sweaty bum.

'They're here!' Robbie squealed, rubbing her hands with glee.

'You beauty, need a couple of creamy climaxes today,' I said licking my lips.

There was a frantic scramble to 'prepare ourselves' for our suitors. Working ladies (certainly in the establishments where I have toiled) were fastidious about intimate hygiene, and we all wanted to be in pristine readiness for our fabulous fire boys. They even wore their uniform when we progressed to the 'spa phase' – it truly does not get much better than this.

Every available bidet was pressed into service – it was like musical chairs, for there weren't enough of these porcelain contraptions to go around the clambering quims. We wanted to be clean before we were *licked* clean. For this was all the fire crew wanted to do. They wanted to munch for so long in the 'downstairs restaurant' that the chairs were metaphorically up on the tables and the lights were out. They were the cunnilingus kings – no prick, all lick – the purveyor of punani – the go-getters of girlee ghee – the captains of cunt and fans of the fanjita.

Boy did they love licking pussy, and we thought all our Valentine's days had come at once. If their spontaneous visit coincided with a rest day the sheer loss was enough to make you want to commit hara kiri (in much the same way that missing the winning goal for England in a world cup would rankle for years after). And God forbid that it should be interrupted by any pyrotechnics. The innate love of one's fellow man would be sorely lacking. Who cared about charred bodies and damage to property when the ultimate fantasy was unfolding.

We formed a circle round a huge bed in the cavernous spa room, our heads touching faintly in the middle and our bodies (and welcoming pussies) pointing to the edge. It was like a sexual Busby Berkley movie. Then they performed.

Hi ho silver and bring it on! Our lovely lads would kneel at the vagina of their chosen goddess, making themselves comfy – for they were in for the long haul. No half-hearted stab at bringing a woman off would do. They took great pride in their service to moll-kind. The chairman of Sony called it the 'total immersion theory'. Whatever your chosen craft or endeavour, be the very best that you can be. They collectively were. Once orgasm(s) were achieved then they would wait to move onto the next grateful furburger.

This was all fine and dandy, but women reach the vinegar stroke at a different rate – and more often than not I was the culprit holding up the revolving restaurant.

'For fuck's sake hurry up, can't you,' the girl to my left would cry, since we always went anti-clockwise.

Now ladies know as well as I do that once concentration is lost you are back in the pit lane to start the race all over again, so complaining is eminently counter productive.

'Shut the fuck up, you dopey cow!' I would snarl, since I had fallen into the verbal ways of my Aussie sisters-in-crime.

This particular situation was illuminated by a conversation I had with a co-worker at another parlour.

'Customer of mine said he saw you the other day and that you was 'hard work' she said

'What does that mean precisely?' I asked.

'Well, he said you took about 15 or 20 minutes to come,' she jeered

'So what if I did?' I huffed 'That's not very long.'

'You dippy cunt, you – I *fake* it in three minutes.'

'Well, its people like you that have made the men folk of today so bloody lazy. If everyone's faking then they lose interest with someone that's really going for gold.'

Talk about being stitched up by your bitches-in-arms.

Back to the Spa room, where the air was full of the noises of *pleasure* (except for the woman on my left). The hour was drawing to a close, and between the eight of us (for there were eight of them) the equivalent of three schooners of jolly juice had been teased from between our trembling legs. Happy days and happy snail-trails of lubricated slabs of silverside. Fire crew arise – I salute you!

The burning question, howeveer, is: would I ever take an Aussie lover? Maybe when my arse learns to plait custard!

Sick
Puppies

If the most popular question from a punter concerns the availability of an uncovered blow-job, the most common question anyone else asks is: 'What's the kinkiest shit you've ever done?'

For the millionth time I reply by rote: 'Define kinky'. If I furnish the interrogators with any information, somewhere along the line it will be used against me in the most judgemental of ways. If a person bombs along a motorway at 130 mph it doesn't inherently make them a racing driver. In the same way, my partaking in some requested activity by a man doesn't make me a pervert. The difference between a flower and a weed is a judgement, and sex workers are up to their flaps in judicators. And audacious sexual antics are not exclusively the province of working ladies.

The most interesting aspect is how a man *knows* that (for example) wearing a gas mask while being plugged anally with the handle of a feather duster will produce the 'eureka' of his sexual life. It's not necessarily something you stumble across accidentally, after all. If space is the final frontier, then man knows no bounds for pushing the sexual envelope. Every vile carnal thought is multiplied billions of times around the world and everyone wants to keep up with the sexy Joneses for fear that they are missing out on something that they have never even conceived before. Conversely, we can congratulate ourselves with the thought that there are people whose imaginations are just as deranged as ours.

Women are well known for discussing the minutiae of all things sexual. My (non-worker) mate Madge the Vadge and I often gabble till the cows come home about sex and its rich tapestry. A few years ago the subject matter was what we fantasised about when we masturbated. Unlike men we not only admit to wanking but also delve into the deep recesses of our minds and share the experience with each other. We confess to the darkest, dankest, depraved thoughts with utter impunity. And we are relieved when someone else admits to feeling the same way about something particularly gross.

'Is it normal to think about dogs when I touch myself?' she asked nervously.

'Depends what breed,' I joked. 'There may be a protected doggie species owned by the Crown that we don't know about – y'know, like swans. Best leave corgis out to be on the safe side.'

'If you aren't going to take this seriously I'm hanging up.'

I cackled like the proverbial hen and replied: 'Of course it's normal. Well at least I do, and loads of my workmates around the world have expressed the same thought or fantasy. I think it's the tongue and the wet, licky, sloppy filthy sound – I'm getting a wide-on talking about it.'

'Oh, thank Christ for that!' she gushed. 'I thought I was strange or something.'

'Didn't they use to have lapdogs for that very purpose years ago, underneath the old crinolines?'

'Don't know, but all I do know is the colour and breed of the bloody thing when I'm having a kit-kat shuffle [woman wank].'

'Let me guess – wouldn't be a black Alsatian by any chance, now would it?' was my rhetorical question.

'How did you know that?' she exclaimed, 'You're freaky.'

'What I don't know about sex and the human condition can be written on the back of postage stamp.'

'So it's not weird. I don't have to go to a psychiatrist to have my sick head examined,' she asked with a palpable relief.

'Well, you'll be in the waiting room a long time 'cos there will be millions ahead of you. A small word though,' I warned. 'Don't mention the dog thing to any of your boyfriends.'

'But you said it was okay and that everyone did it.'

'Yes, but men are so bloody stupid and literal that the last person I told came marching up the stairs looking so pleased with himself because he'd borrowed a mate's dog – he wanted to make my dreams come true.'

'You're having a laugh.'

'Nope, it's name was Foggy, after the superbike champion. The stupid bloke had driven it all the way from London.'

'What did you do?'

'Gave the poor thing a bowl of water and told the bloke to fuck off.'

Men, eh? Can't live with them and can't tell them intimate secrets lest they get hold of completely the wrong end of the doggie stick. He looked so disappointed (the man not the dog).

I remember vividly a mate of mine telling me about a man who adored being defiled by rent boys. He only chose those who could excrete perfectly hard large stools (now there's a talent – got to be a niche market, but there's probably a call for it somewhere in this twisted world). He would ask them to 'perform' and would rescue the floater from the toilet bowl and wrap it in cling film or tin foil (I am truly not making this up). He would then stick it in the freezer compartment of his fridge. Later when the mood took him, he would unwrap the frozen stool and *insert it up his own anus.* Then he would wait to excrete somebody else's poo at his leisure. Nice! I'm glad I don't get invited to his place for supper: there's no telling what would inadvertently be served for dessert.

Things of a lavatorial nature have always been a source of excitement and intrigue to the British, no more so than with one of my favourite patrons. Daddy Bear (a 20-stone skinhead) was always thinking of ways to spice up his love life, so I should not have been surprised when he puffed visibly with pride on his way up the stairs with his purchases du jour. Seems he had a field day with his bit of retail therapy at Halfords (bikes and auto shops). He toted a veritable cornucopia of plastic tubing and some convoluted funnel attachments.

'And what, pray, am I supposed to do with that?' I asked in a tone of bemusement.

'I want you to piss up my ring piece,' he replied animatedly.

He had worked out the slight 'engineering problem' with his purchased bits and bobs. Varying sizes and colours of funnels and tubing could be constructed so that while I relieved myself in one end it would flow into his freckle. Plus, as an added bonus, he could *see* it happening because the material was clear. He could not have been more pleased with himself had he bought me champagne and chocolates.

Necessity is the mother of invention. Once I had successfully performed I decided to suggest a wild finish.

As he lay on his back in my bath with the warmth of my urine sloshing around inside his rectum, I suggested he very gingerly stand up and let the amber nectar flow back down the tubing , reasoning that by leaning forward he would be able to drink it as well. He was thrilled that I was truly entering into the spirit of the proceedings. I now have the mental image of this scene whenever I have hiccups, as drinking from the opposite side of glass is my favoured way of dealing with it.

Same bathroom, different man. Step forward Supernerd – the epitome of computer geek with a touch of the ever-prevalent Mr Bean thrown in. His predilection was extraordinarily interesting, and was probably the easiest £100 I have ever had to earn in my colourful life. All I had to do was put the plug in the bath and turn the cold tap on. I didn't have to be in any specific uniform or sexy underwear. In fact, so early was his call one morning that it was jim-jams and cold cream.

I didn't have to touch him, either. All I had to do was watch in an imperious manner. He would undress in the bedroom and emerge wearing a pair of *green wellington boots* and a look of rapture on his face. He would climb into the bath with an air of excitement that caused him to tremble. He stood perfectly still and stared at me intently while I returned his gaze, thinking to myself 'Do not laugh; do not laugh'. As the level of water got closer to the rim of his wellies tears sprang to his eyes. He did not at any time touch himself but his dick would burgeon to elephantine proportions.

Then the miracle would happen. As the cold water splashed into his boots he would simultaneously come. Very bloody clever stuff, if you ask me. The human psyche is so infinitely fascinating and he was very generous in explaining how this sexual quirk had become the *only* thing that could get him off in this way.

'My mother and sisters used to go fishing at the local river. I was about ten at the time. It was just after my birthday on St. Patrick's Day and mum bought these green wellington boots.'

'So you were coming to sexual fruition at the time?' I enquired, getting to grips with my new role as psycho/sexual counsellor.

'Yes, you could say that. Anyway, it was uncommonly hot for March and we went to hunt for tadpoles and suchlike. There were other groups of people there and one woman was taking off her top. As I watched, her bra snapped to reveal these beautiful breasts and at that moment a boat that had passed by made the river swell sufficiently to make the cold water trickle into my boots. I've never forgotten it, and it's now the only trigger which allows me to come. You've been very understanding about it.'

'Are you saying that in your own computer speak an Ingram has been created and you are now programmed to come only that way?' I asked.

'No it's just that I don't *want* to come any other way, and you have been charitable enough to allow me to do so, so I thank you from the bottom of my heart.'

Well it's nice to be appreciated, and I guess he would be hard pressed to find a regular girlfriend of the Laura Ashley variety to accommodate his penchant for water and wellies. At times like these I feel I am doing something worthwhile that contributes to my personal growth, and it's a hell of a story to tell at dinner parties.

One character who has no trouble finding a willing victim for his outrageous penchants is a personal mate of mine called Nick. How he clicks into these women is truly beyond me, for it's not as if he's a part French and bunk up man. His particular bent is about control (his tenure in the armed services having not been entirely wasted), and I have seen it up close and personal.

I introduced him to a girlfriend of mine since they were both single and looking for a soul mate. She had a 'power job' in the city and was a very self-contained formidable woman. We met in her luxurious suite at the grand hotel for convivial drinkies prior to an evening meal. She was dressed in a tight halter- top and slightly flared mini skirt. This is how the date unfolded:

'Take your panties off right now,' he ordered.

As an opening gambit to a potentially hot blind-date I thought in was a little tasteless and motioned to him to meet me outside the bathroom door.

'What the fuck do you think you're playing at?' I hissed.

'Trust me,' he replied coolly 'I know what I'm doing.'

She very obediently did as she was bid and we set off along a very blustery Brighton seafront. Her short skirt very tantalisingly was almost (but not quite) revealing all her bits. She must have felt very vulnerable and exposed. Nick strode ahead dispassionately like some sheik with his many wives.

Upon being seated at our chosen restaurant, Pru got up again stating that she needed to go to the loo.

'Sit down,' he snapped.

She made a half-hearted show of whining about it but did as she was told. Nick made sure that the three-course meal was eaten *as slowly as possible* to create the maximum discomfort. We eventually left and Pru pleaded: 'If I don't go now I'm going to wet myself.'

'Then please do so,' he said.

She started to retreat to a hidden alley when he barked: 'Just do it here' – 'here' being a busy, well-lit Brighton street exposed to hundreds of cars and people. And she did. She straddled the edge of the pavement and gushed down her bare legs. Nick looked on scornfully while I wondered what kind of twilight zone I had the pleasure of encountering.

'I suppose you think you can go and change at the hotel now pretty miss. Well think again, we're going to have a few more drinks.' And we did. Her humiliation and subjugation was complete and I didn't hear one word of true complaint from her.

Eventually we arrived back at her hotel suite where he decided, for his final command, to change her from a she to an 'it'.

'Strip, get in the corner of the room and bend over' he ordered. He then lifted a lampshade from elsewhere in the room, placed it over her head – and ordered more champagne.

When I spoke to her the next day I steeled myself to ask how she was and how the evening had finished up.

'I just had the best time. Where on earth did you find such a sexy man?'

'Known him for ages, but I didn't know he was quite like *that*,' I replied with relief.

I then rang him to get his side of the tawdry story.

'It was quite a good evening,' he drawled in a lazy 'I've had better' manner.

'Good evening?' I thundered, 'You can't even *pay* for that kind of date.'

'I get women like that all the time,' he replied absent mindedly.

'How did you know she would respond to you in that way and not haul off and slug you right in your self-satisfied face,' I asked.

'Because you working ladies haven't cornered the market in perversity and I have always been able to find a woman willing to do whatever I want them to.'

'But,' I protested, 'you're so extreme.'

'You may think so my friend, but plenty of your sisterhood help keep my powder dry. Some of them are so "out there" that I have to finish the relationship because they're too sick and twisted.'

'Like what, for example?' I asked.

'Once a girl wrote me an entire script of the things that she wanted us to do for kicks, and as I read on I felt more repulsed – she wanted us to get a transit van and actually scout around for a young hitchhiker to kidnap and do God knows what to her before we released her.'

'I think you made the right judgment call – maybe you're not so fucked in the head after all,' I said.

'You might think not when I tell you what I did with my current partner the other night.'

I feigned lack of interest but was dying to know what it was he deemed noteworthy enough to mention is dispatches.

'I had her trussed and dangling from a tree in the meadows at the back of my country cottage – and then I went to the pub.'

'She let you do this? Wasn't she cold – didn't you worry about her?'

'Nope, what's to worry about? As for being cold, who cares?'

I swear he must have a loving compassionate bone somewhere in his wiry leather clad (he rides extremely fast bikes) body. He imparted to me the rest of his romantic evening *à deux*.

On his return, mercifully, she was still alive – had neither hanged herself nor been eaten by foxes. Then he tied her to the trunk of another tree and whipped her till she passed into semi consciousness. I am assuming this was the conclusion of the 'foreplay' part of the evening. He carried her to his cottage while she was still in her comatose state and pushed some stinging nettles he had thoughtfully gathered into her front and back botty. Say what you like about our Nick, he truly is at one with nature.

She came round to find herself spread-eagled on the robust oak kitchen table. Her outer labia had been smeared with jam (again, I am not making this up) and he had found an inquisitive neighbour's dog to enter into this night of dubious bridled passion. Even this was not enough, for she tarried downstairs long after Nick had got bored and hit the sleeping sack. She finished herself off with a red-hot poker from the Aga cooker.

Hell of a date. It had all the elements that are missing from the love lives of so many people – excitement, pain, expectation, degradation, terror – and so many marks that would take some time to heal. And to think I so narrowly missed out on this esoteric treatment. Were it not for the fact I was going to the theatre one evening, he had designs on coming round and 'putting me through my paces' Thank God for the stage show 'Blues Brothers'. Maybe someone is watching over us.

I will conclude my discourse on all things sinister and most unnerving with Steve, a perfectly normal, indeed handsome man, who, once in my flat, wishes to play out various fantasies. So far, so good. By the time he has been cantilevered into bra stockings and lace panties his face is contorted into a prepubescent teenager. His toes point into the luxurious silk of the fashioned and seamed hosiery which has been purloined from yours truly His voice changes to that of a conglomeration of the scariest movies ever made and he talks like a little scared girlie. It is truly puke making.

Stage left enters me as – Rosemary West (his idea, *definitely not mine*). I went with this sick flow (more verbal than anything else, I hasten to add) and wondered whether press reporting of heinous crimes should be somewhat curtailed. I realise that reading and re-enacting are two different things, but plant a seed in some people's minds and they will morph into mega-unsavoury.

As usual I take it all in my stride. It takes a lot to shock me (like an Englishman actually proffering a gratuity!) If I were an ice cream I would be plain vanilla and it would *not* find its way smeared all over the voluptuous folds of my body. No, that would be a waste – it would be devoured with relish.

To me, anything else would be unnatural.

Travels With My C(a)unt
Part 1

T hey say wherever you roam you take yourself with you. You can't run away from your unhappiness – you can only inevitably experience more. That's life. Having travelled extensively and with great hope I have inadvertently stumbled across the differing attitudes to sex and sexual relationships. Sometimes this starts at the airport.

Heathrow, and everyone travelling looks decidedly jumpy. Lockerbie and various other air disasters are fresh in all the travellers' minds. We have our luggage scanned and step forward – -a likely lad (if memory serves me, a Singapore Airlines security manager) doing his best to put my mind off what, let's face it, could be a fatal journey. Mr Security, all peaked cap and knowing stare, engages in thinly veiled banter, and 15 minutes later I spy him nonchalantly flicking through books in the departures section of the airport.

He does a double take of 'raspberry' (the alternative Oscars) proportions and I decide to play. 'Come to mommie bear,' I think, 'because there will only be one winner.'

We have vile airport coffee and prepare to duel under the frenetic atmosphere that embodies most airports. A broom cupboard is suggested for a convenient bit of duty-freak shopping. I decline. My contraceptive pill is ensconced safely in my luggage, which is at this moment being transferred to the plane and, besides, I can't do it standing up. Yes, I know they do it in the movies, but show me a man who can not only lift, but also *fuck*, while lifting a 13-stone woman and I'll start believing in leprechauns. I can never see at rock concerts much less get my tits out for the lead singer, since no-one is strong enough to put me on his shoulders without carrying life-long injuries.

It's easy to be an opportunist in the heady atmosphere of aviation fuel and incomprehensible tannoy systems. My flight was once delayed for 15 hours in Bangkok. It was highly inconvenient since I hadn't really slept much for the preceding two days. The previous day (having spent all my holiday money in Penang) I had spent 24 hours wondering how I would spin out my 'two free drinks vouchers at the Dusit thanni Hotel'. I went to the bar to see if there were any likely lads that might want to buy this little cupie doll a blow-out evening meal.

I prepared to do battle in the luxurious cocktail bar, so being perfectly coiffed and, with a little black dress adorning and caressing my freshly ice-cubed nipples, I sought out my knight in shining armour. I walked slap-bang into an Elvis convention! Luckily for me they were out of the normal white jump suit kit, and mega lucky was I that most of them came from America and treated English ladies like queens. I was ma'am this and ma'am that and was being bought drinks with offer of a meal later. God, I'm good. Hit 'em up, move 'em out!

My date for the evening also had a penchant like my own for heavy rock/metal. It was like a Cyclops finding another person with a third eye. I was in hog heaven, gorging stupendous food overlooking a smog/pollution filled Bangkok from a revolving restaurant and discussing the merits of the individual lead singers from Deep Purple. Due to extreme lassitude I wasn't feeling in the least bit horny. I was so tired I could have cried. My nipples are normally the gateway of feeling to my pudenda, but giving them a few preliminary strokes to see how the land was lying I discovered that I was literally dead from the neck down. Why, my inner and outer labia were barely on speaking terms at all.

Mr Midwest America was unfazed and gave me *six hours of uninterrupted oral*. Had I not needed to catch a flight back to Sydney I'm sure another six would have been on the menu., but this Elvis had left the building.

It was 6.30 am and Bangkok airport revealed that a 15-hour delay would be our fate. (To think I left a stupendous polish for this.) We were herded to a unprepossessing grey concrete building posing as an airport motel and was told this was our temporary home for the next 12 hours. Nothing to do but flirt: no rest for the mega-wicked. I spotted my quarry and began circling to get closer to the meat of the matter. He didn't stand a chance. It wasn't a fair contest.

Over breakfast we swapped glances and room numbers. By lunchtime we were touching one another and telling each other our condensed life histories and innermost precious secrets with the promise of a bit of afternoon delight. His knock at my door late in the afternoon had more frisson that a Mr Sparky. We lay in each other's arms, stroking, caressing and kissing. He massaged me and I resisted the urge to fall asleep because something was stirring in the valley below – I had a wide-on the size of the Grand Canyon. This was going to be good. 'Come on train,' I thought.

We started to maul each other with great passion borne of a 9-hour courtship/foreplay. Then disaster occurred. A knock at the door told us that the plane had arrived earlier than anticipated and was in fact ready for us at the airport and would we please (pretty please, with sugar on top) make our way as quickly as possible to the lobby where a coach would escort us. We had travelled so far on this journey of excitement and rampant sexuality we felt damn cheated at the prospect of doing it as a quick zipless fuck. If you spend hours lovingly preparing a cordon bleu meal you can't wolf it standing up. We clung to each other in despair. I pressed myself so hard into his body, wanting to climb inside him. He reacted likewise. For the first and probably only time in my life *I came by just dry humping.* In fact we both did, a glorious simultaneous combustion of our loins. How perfectly splendid.

We shared the same flight to Australia but didn't sit together. It was a complete love affair with a beginning, middle and very fast end, simply perfect in its symmetry. I never saw him again.

Why is it that we always meet Mr Right at the airport, or is it that intoxicating atmosphere of trains, boats and planes that makes us cleave, with every fibre of our being, to Mr. Right Now? I went to some charlatan soothsayer many moons ago, which is something many people do when they are unhappy. She told me I would meet Mr Tall, Dark, Handsome, hung like a moose, mega wedged up, blah blah blah vomit. But what hooked me was that I would meet him at the baggage reclaim of an *unspecified* foreign airport, and the key to this kismet was that we would both be gunning for the same bag. My luggage at the time consisted of the whole side of a cow skin complete with leather tits and horns, so I found the prospect highly improbable. Try matching that. The premise was (due to the nature of my 'shrinking violet taste') nigh on impossible – but, optimist and romantic fool that I am, I bought it anyway.

How many air miles I clocked up searching for this bloke would be hard to fathom, but there were a lot of noughts. Likewise zero regarding my hero. Not only was I tempting fate, I was lifting my skirt and inviting it to bugger me. 'Perhaps I should just buy another bag,' I thought, but that would be cheating the system. 'Why stop there?' was my next gloomy thought 'Why not have a complete personality transplant and physical makeover – rejig and totally reconfigure the thought processes and ideals which have shaped you into what you are today?'

This was getting complicated. Hard enough to find a man who played the kind of tunes that make your soul stir and your ears bleed, let alone one who stowed his sacred cow in the hold. Then the miracle happened. Changi Airport, Singapore, spotlessly clean and functional (unlike many cocks I have encountered) offered up a burning bush of sorts. Okay, so I bent the rules slightly – his luggage was carry-on, it being the most stupendous briefcase I had ever seen. The handle was fashioned from the horns of the beast and there were tits on the underbelly. Fuck me! My legs turned to jelly and my bowels turned to water. Thank God I had washed my hair and was looking post-Lankowi Island 'tanned top totty'. We were on the same flight, and unbeknown to him he had a stalker. I saw the ground staff label his luggage 'All the Way to Gatwick' and knew by virtue of the queue we formed that we were both travelling first class.

'You never know,' I thought licking my lips lasciviously 'the Mile-high Club may be in for a surprise new application.' Women make great spies I decided, and I kept him in close range and studied him from afar. He did not appear to be love's young dream , but maybe that's where I had it wrong for so long. 'Looks don't matter,' people say. Well they bloody well matter to me! Henry Kissinger used to end up bedding half the glamorous females on this planet, and let's face it chums, even the oil would recoil from a proposed painting of the fella.

No, my man would be dynamic yet sensitive, a real go-getter and achiever, someone to look up to and someone to watch over me. I could learn to love a squat overweight young man with a gargantuan nose. We boarded and ,yes, as if our stars were inter-twined and twinned we were in the same row. Let the games commence!

I struggled outrageously to put my duty free in the overhead compartment. He didn't move a muscle. 'Pig,' I thought – an inauspicious start to the romance of the century. 'How can I think that of my destiny and my intended?' I reasoned in desperation. I had nabbed the window seat and effusively said: 'Excuse me'. The pig again did not move. I clamoured indelicately over the top of him and thought that the chances of me ever doing this to him while naked (or even *wanting* to, since I don't do rude) were dwindling, as my dream receded into the Asian sky.

He rebuffed all of my advances with studied indifference. He would not engage in conversation or anything else. I had been through my entire 'go girl' repertoire but this fish didn't want to bite. I felt like screaming 'Look, you dozy sod, this fortune-teller told me about you and we're supposed to romance and live happily ever after. You are ruining the fantasy.' But for once in my life I stayed silent.

Bombay turned to Bahrain then to Frankfurt and as we descended we met the cold grey wet clouds that herald most people's arrival into England. At baggage reclaim we stood fairly close together, since the outrageous tariff for first class ensured that at least our luggage arrived before the plebs. Faint heart never won fair lady, so I summoned what was left of my battered self-esteem and approached this forbidding man.

'I'm so sorry to trouble you, but would you mind telling me where you got that fabulous brief case – it reminds me so much of my own luggage.'

As if on cue my cow appeared on the conveyor belt to much hilarity from the assembled crowd.

For the first time in the entire journey he allowed himself a faint smile and replied: 'It's not my briefcase, its my cousin's. He left it to me in his will and I've just come back from his funeral – sorry I haven't been very chatty.'

He surveyed my eclectic choice in baggage and in bidding me goodbye said: 'You two would have made a good pair.'

To say I was a stunned mullet would be pretty fair. Oh Lord, why don't you just gaze upon a soul in agony. Over before it began. Fated to roam this earth for my other half forever because he's dead already. You can't love a corpse, and I had no memory to keep me warm at night. Torn bloody testicles and boil infested bums!

They say our creator (if you believe in the Genesis theory) is all-seeing, all-knowing, so it follows that he has seen me having far too much of a good time. The premature death of my intended (according to the white witch) was somehow supposed to stop me in my tracks.

'If I can't be with the one I was *supposed* to love,' I thought stoically, 'then I'll just love the one I'm with at the time. Football teams have substitutes, doctors have locums and I shall have to content myself with option two.' You can't keep a good woman down.

Phucket Airport on route to Kho Samui. I had a hangover that would have killed a pig. I dimly remembered playing air guitar the previous evening with a long haired Thai hippie, who seemed like a good choice of local takeaway for the evening, in a music bar full of Thai prostitutes and the ugliest of motherfuckers from all around the world. The music wasn't bad either: Black Sabbath, Jimi Hendrix, Faith no More, Chilli peppers . . . oh, and of course Deep Purple. It was great to be in this type of place because all the guys were trying to hit on the diminutive 'lotus blossoms' and left me the hell alone which was just how I wanted it. I passed out with my willing hippie victim only to find upon waking (or should that be coming to) that thousands of baht had mysteriously disappeared from my money belt. I looked in his trouser pockets (we women are trained for this covert action, and we spy with extreme prejudice), to find the same amount had transferred itself via osmosis to him. Bloody cheek! I woke him up and asked him what he was playing at. He had lost his command of the English language overnight (along it seems with my money) and stood sheepishly listening to my tirade. I couldn't trade the ultimate insult of telling him what a dud fuck he was since I couldn't remember a thing, and frankly if he had been intent upon robbing me then I hoped I hadn't. What I did remember was that there was no tacit understanding of a financial agreement being entered.

Seems a rather circuitous route to being a gigolo – why not just ask? Kerb crawling is one thing, ambulance chasing another, but this was beyond the pale. If MacDonalds force-fed passers-by with a quarter pounder and charged for the privilege it would-be mentioned is despatches. Only in Asia can the payee become the payer. Thailand *is* a country whose great pulling power is sex (or marriage) for sale, but it becomes complex where female travellers are concerned. On their part (the would be service providers) the thought that we want to pay for sexual services is an ignorant and erroneous assumption based on the fact that one is white, seemingly single (or without a chaperone) and over 21. Those are the criteria. Therefore in their mind you must be gagging for it, and they see marketing/no-strings sex opportunity. We are supposed to be so grateful that we would give them enough to buy a small house.

I have bought a male escort in Asia a couple of times. Why? Because I could. I went to a club that had male dancers miming to varying songs but mainly the Weather Girls' 'It's raining men'. It was terrific entertainment and at the end one could choose, for a fee, which gentleman one would like to go home with. Perversely I was not interested in the body, nor if the guy in question had a rudimentary knowledge of the English language. I wanted a bloke with a bike, so that he could ride with me round Phuket Island. It seemed cheaper than hiring a motorbike and the clincher was that I could fuck but not ride anyway. This promised much more fun. At the end of the evening I motioned to the Poppa-san that I'd like some come-company. Communication in our native language didn't seem to be getting us anywhere, so I used that time-honoured technique of sign language.

What I thought was a pretty good impersonation of a motorbike being revved up via the handles somehow was translated as, (since my jerking wrists were 20 inches apart) me wanting to wank a Thai national with an unusually large penis. Much nervous giggling ensued as they wondered where they were going to find a guy of elephantine proportions at such short notice: they hate to lose a juicy business deal. I added another piece of body miming – that of a foot, kick-starting a moped. Nope, that made them even more panic-stricken. I looked like a wild stallion stamping its hoof. One of the dancers whispered to another something like: 'want man hung like horse'.

There goes any aspiration of being a sign language teacher. A bilingual bystander with much mopping of brow and sighing of relief resolved the misunderstanding. I choose my man.

It's a strange thing, but if one works in the sex industry one doesn't want to give the 'bought-boy' a hard time. In fact you go out of your way to make them feel comfortable and strain to be as undemanding as possible when technically they should be doing this very thing for you. It's a hell of a double whammy.

I was perfectly contented with my sightseeing around the island, being chauffeured by this handsome young man, and made a great deal out of gesticulating to him that 'This is my bed and that is yours.' This wasn't good enough for him. He had been trained like Pavlov's dog to paint by numbers, play it by the book and expect the 'farrang' to be rapacious and mega sexual. So this customer could not waive her right to sex and would jolly well have to have it. 'Okay' I thought, 'if I must.'. Make that a triple whammy then: you either end up with a hooker you haven't asked for, or a fuck that you hadn't planned on.

My second male hooker was purchased in Singapore. I needed a dinner companion to meet a co-worker and her boyfriend who had been circumnavigating the world in the proceeding months (what jet set lives we led). His name was Kelvin aka Onassis. He was an astonishingly good-looking man. We made a great fraction – he was half my age. He was Malay, and a curious hybrid of Christian and Islam.The problem was he was *too* good-looking. I have a little rule: never make love with a man who is better looking than one self. Of course I rescind this rule when it suits me with borderline cases, but I was adamant it was dinner and polite chit-chat only. Things couldn't have gone better.

Consequently whenever I flew into Changi in following years he would always greet me in full silk national costume and insisted that I save hotel charges and stay with him. This was because whenever I took him back to my bullshit five-star deluxe, Orchard Road, over airconditioned hotel, the doorman would routinely stop us on the suspicion that a *prostitute* was entering. The fact that he had the wrong prostitute was a source of great amusement or irritation, depending on the way we were feeling at the time.

Airports, you name them – I have surely buried my head in the chest of the conquest, snared from my departure party, with the Clash anthem/jingle 'Should I stay or should I go?' swirling in my mind.

Men are not above this heightened ardour or sentiment based on imminent departure. While having a relaxing gin and tonic at the Dynasty hotel I spied another 'must have'. It transpired that he had been watching me from afar and had made up *his* mind *my* arse (or any other part of my anatomy) was his. He was due to leave Singapore four hours later and, as usual, the sexual tension was so heightened as to be insurmountable. Tickets were changed, holiday plans rearranged. Travel and mini adventures go hand in hand. Why is it one can always get laid abroad but within 24 hrs of arriving home it's back to hot chocolate and cold wanking lube?

I know gay guys that deliberately set out on a rail journey to see who they can snare, like an ultimate 'have it away day'. Yes it's the travelling hopefully rather than the arrival that's the key, and if life is what happens when you're making plans then don't waste that fertile time of abandonment worrying about what's going to happen when you get there, for you could be blinded to the glorious romance and intrigue of the journey.

Travels With My C(a)unt

Part 2

A patron of mine (who is a judge) made a very thought provoking statement the other day. In all his years sitting on the bench, he told me, 'I have noticed one thing time and time again – that is how different women are in the north and the south of the country'

'You mean sexually?' I replied.

'No, in their attitude to men. I have found that women in the north of England don't mind being hit by their husbands but will not put up with infidelity, while the women in the south don't mind their husband being unfaithful but don't like to be hit.'

Illuminating and riveting stuff. It takes all sorts to make a world and I have encountered most of them along the way. Dr Spock (of Star Trek rather than baby fame) would find it all most sublime and fascinating. That takes care of the north and south but how about more globally east and west?

Given that Penang in Malaysia is divided up into at least four nationalities, many religions and ethnicity, then attitudes (and in some cases mind boggling ignorance) is encountered on a daily basis. As for sex, it's a veritable quagmire of bigotry and misinformation. A perfect example was my friend Sheik. He was a Muslim and married with four children, and you could always rely upon seeing him drinking and womanising away the steamy Malaysian nights at various locations in Georgetown.

We started talking one night about the death penalty which had been imposed on two stupid Australian men who had smuggled drugs into the country despite clear warnings of the punishment posted at all the airports. Sheik worked at Penang prison and kept me posted as to how the process was unfolding. We became firm friends.

'Sheik,' I once asked, 'I'm slightly familiar with the Koran and I feel sure this 20 pints-a-night-and-floosies thing is verboten.'

'Ver *what*?'

'It's not allowed, pal.'

'Ah!' he exclaimed. 'The interpretation that I have is, as long as I can still speak my name or 'tidat mabo' as they say in bhasa Malay – which means 'I am not drunk' – then its permissible.'

'Oh well, that's okay then,' I cooed facetiously. 'And the women? I mean, your strike rate is better than Pele himself.'

'I always preferred George Best, but to answer your question is very simple. If I am going to see another woman then I make sure my wife is satisfied before I leave the house.'

'You have an answer for every day of the week,' I said smiling with incredulity 'You're just being very selective with your interpretation so that you can limbo dance under the tenets of your faith.'

As an afterthought I added: 'Do you ever say to the missus 'Hurry up and come ,you mongrel ,I'm late for a date with my girlfriend?"

He didn't get angry or agitated at my relentless questioning and gentle teasing: he had squared it in his mind with the prophet Mohammed and this naturally gave him carte blanche to fornicate to his devout Muslim heart's content. He neatly deflected the conversation away from his lack of devotion to his god, and the abundance of freelance 'prawn' by asking: 'Who's your lover at the moment, then?'

'Amerjeet. Sikh Indian – head doorman at the Shangri-la,' I replied.

'What's he like in bed?'

'That's what I don't get. I don't know if its an Indian thing or a Sikh thing because I've never had one before, but he just devours all the knowledge of what turns me on and does it perfectly every time like its an exam or something. It's weirdly impersonal, just like performing surgery.'

'It's probably something to do with the Karma Sutra culture'.

'Mmm,' I replied thoughtfully. 'Don't think I'll see him for much longer, though. When we check into a motel I feel like a whore.'

'I thought you *were* in Australia.'

'Well I'm not in Australia now and I'm off duty for the foreseeable future – this is for fun.'

I spotted his girlfriend in the sweaty rock club and bade him farewell because I needed to get some sleep before the mosque, which was adjacent to my guest house, started pumping out the call to prayer on their loudspeakers. Since wild rock music is *my* religion I wondered how conciliatory the reaction would be were I to blast out AC/DC at five in the morning. How come Islam has got round the noise abatement problem? Maybe this bloke Mohammed had a swift word to those in the know.

I had an 18-month 'lost weekend' in Penang, and for most of that time languished and often moped in a small 'kampong' located on the waterfront in Batu Ferringhi. My life's blueprint had gone most disastrously askew. All of the money I had amassed by gruelling hard yakka in Australia had had been 'misappropriated' by some thieving bastard conman who resided on the Gold Coast, which is the Aussie equivalent of our very own 'Costa del crime'. I was crushed, and spent a lot of my days in what was supposed to be paradise, in a 'poor me what have I done to deserve this?' haze. One of the visitors at the guesthouse said to me one day, 'You should be grateful and happy.'. I asked this diminutive Chinaman from Ipoh how he arrived at this absurd notion.

'If you didn't have any money you wouldn't have any thing to worry about, and now you have had the money taken away you are therefore liberated from that worry.'

To laugh or to cry, that is the question. These Chinese blokes have got a Zen-like attitude in spades. No wonder there are so many revered philosophers in that neck of the woods. It didn't make me feel better, but I consoled myself that I would be celebrating Gung Hei Fat Choy (Chinese New Year) with a date from Kuala Lumpur.

He had stayed at the Ah Beng guest house before, and on each subsequent visit had greeted me with the words 'are you still here?' I stifled the urge to tell him I was in fact struggling with either clinical depression or a mild nervous breakdown and was rooted aimlessly and listlessly to the spot. Men don't want you when you are ill and don't like you moaning, since they like to monopolise that particular market. We are here to please and to nurture, and in return they fuck us (badly) and buy a few dinners.

And that dinner, or should I say banquet, was tonight. It was a pleasant evening (yummy food and mind bogglingly bad sex, but time well spent) and I felt my soul was on the long road to recovery. We sat under a huge tree in front of the guesthouse and watched the vista of seashore and brightly shining stars. It was three in the morning and all was well when we heard soft footsteps approaching round the rough dirt track which passed as the Kampong road.

It was a local musician with his guitar slung over his back, and trotting behind him was Keidi the dog, so named because it had been imprisoned and the village had collectively rescued it and welcomed it into the fold.

There was only one lamp in the whole of the village, and as Keidi passed she cocked her leg and did the usual. A lamppost is a lamppost in any language. The musician turned back to the dog, looked furtively to the left and to the right and proceeded to drop his trousers.

My date and I gazed on in rapt fascination. We could not move or speak since this unfolding scene had hijacked us. I thought it was a bit out of order to squat and take a dump on the path, but hey, we've all been caught short. What followed next was of puke-making proportions. His squat turned to a kneeling on all fours position and his bottom pouted and *was proffered to the dog*. Not only did Keidi take the bait, licking and lapping willingly, but also, disconcertingly, he (the dog) appeared to have been *trained* to do so.

It wasn't all one sided – the musician was not a selfish lover. He had the presence of mind to give his doggie a reach around and was lovingly stroking Keidi's cock. Bile rose in our throats as we watched this study in bestiality. I wondered whether Keidi would have preferred to stay a prisoner. There's an English advert for pet food which goes 'Nine out of ten owners said their pets preferred it.' Oh dear, through the gloom we could clearly see what this pet liked, and this was just foreplay, for Mr Kombaya gently led his 'Gung Hei Fat Choy special' down to the seashore for part two of this canine coupling. I don't know which of the protagonists got anally fucked or sucked but there was a lot of barking going on.

That morning I went to the local hairdresser/gambling house/coffee shop/cafe for a spot of breakfast. The headline in the local newspaper was: BEWARE ALL WHITE TOURISTS, AIRLINE WORKERS, HAIRDRESSERS, ACTORS AND FASHION HOUSE WORKERS AND DANCERS. Perceived wisdom was that anyone vaguely associated with these professions and/or fitting the bill as a traveller was riddled with that modern day plague, Aids. After what I had seen a few hours earlier (before the damn mosque woke me up), that particular ignorant pronouncement was the least of their worries. Stupidity irritates me, but stupidity based on disinformation really makes my blood boil. Its like old wives' tales.

A lady standing at a bus stop in Georgetown got chatting to me one day and admitted that she had not washed her hair for 70 days after the birth of her first child. She saw my look of horror and explained that her mother had taught her that to put water on the head sooner than 100 days after the birth would result in great sickness. How can one disabuse a trusting soul of that notion especially when it has been handed down through the ages from mother to child? Try breaking that little chain of belief.

I read the paper with barely contained rage. In horror and retaliation I found the words tumbling unbidden from my mouth to nobody in particular: 'We may be what you so laughingly call the infidel but at least we don't train our pets to feltch our ring piece!'

Mr Chang, the owner of the illustrious establishment enquired politely what the heck I was talking about. I told him what I had seen and he laughed it off with a dismissive 'You too much gin last night'. I couldn't get my dinner date to corroborate my story since he had fled back to Kuala Lumpur, presumably to throw up in the safety of his own bathroom at the memory of his date from hell. So now I was a ferringi [foreigner] fantasist with a drink problem, and no amount of arguing could turn their mindset around.

A few days passed and I finally emerged from my 18 months' fog of despair. I decided, just for the hell of it, to say 'yes' to all the beach boys who had ever propositioned me during my stay. After all, I never had to see them again and the boredom of perpetually speaking pidgin English and putting up with the stupid attitudes of dire lovers was beginning to put me off the entire male population of the world.

The beach boys were nothing more than glorified male prostitutes. They harboured pretensions of being gym instructor this and sailing instructor that, but a year and a half of observing their way of life made me stay the hell away. They swaggered with their own pathetic self-importance, based on the fact that they 'serviced' some of the less attractive women from all over the world. I had never seen them with a stunner, and wondered if (in the same way that English people think all Asian people look the same) they couldn't tell shit from shinola. I still assume they made am exception in my case.

They had more front than Harrods, and thought they made the relentless arrival of fresh female meat from all corners of the globe feel 'special'. Since 20 plane-loads a day slammed down onto the airport runway there was plenty of raw material to work through. One Valentine's Day a 'dick for hire' guy asked me to post some cards to all of his 'girlfriends' around the world as he was late for a scheduled boat trip. There was a pile of 50 tokens of love and each one contained some spurious story of having lost wages in the sea, of grandmother needing urgent costly medical attention and every old chestnut you have ever heard from a person on the make. Most of these poor unfortunates (women) believed it when the guys said they missed and adored them. There's a sucker born every minute and most of them literally came to suck a bit of exotic black (since most were Malay) cock.

What these women got out of it is beyond my powers of comprehension. They would service these conceited bums and pay for the privilege. They saved for years to make enough, not only for the holiday but to pay for every meal/drink/club/disco and whatever piece of apparel the boy demanded. It was quite a sad spectacle, especially when a lady made a return visit and couldn't find the promised object of her affections.

'What are you doing cowering behind that boat?' I once asked one of the most prolific 'service providers'.

'Me hiding – last year she very beautiful, now she is so big, matcham gaja!'

'What you mean, she's put on weight? But she's probably been saving for a long time to see you, Mo [short for Mohammed],' I replied gravely. 'You can't let her down now – she'll have been looking forward to it.'

'Me no see her, me no sexy for her,' he wailed.

And he spent the rest of the week avoiding this overweight woman. From *her* point of view I would have thought this was just as well, and a terrific result, given that the Malay tongue was never exercised in the total manner to which certainly I had become accustomed. Or should I put this another way: Malay men (along with negros) do not give head.

'How can you make that statement if you haven't had *all* the black men or *all* the Malay men in the world?' a friend once asked.

'I am not prepared to number crunch. The odds are woeful. Stop splitting hairs: I've had loads of both, and based on the my extensive research there is a 100 per cent rate failure rate. I don't fancy the odds and I'm not going to waste my time looking for a good lick if the statistics are stacked against me. Life's too short. They're crap in the sack.'

My wild theory in this regard is due to the fact that in many African and/or Islamic countries the barbaric practice of cliterectomy still flourishes and therefore the guys know there is nothing of nerve-ending quality to lick. Time and motion studies notwithstanding, it's a great time saver. If the entire female population of the world had this small but perfectly formed procedure then it would knock nine-tenths off the time it took a man to 'have an empty', as they wouldn't be required to have a stab at the arcane science of cunnilingus. Conversely, if a matriarchal society issued the edict to chop cock, the freed-up 'head time' would allow us to maybe run the world. (Just a little flight of fancy.)

Another theory is that they regard the experience as unclean or 'non-halal', but in an effort to make it more palatable, being garrotted, hung for three weeks and desiccated is not my idea of a wild time.

I strolled along Batu Ferringhi beach and when the guys came scudding across the waves in their speed boats/jet skies, with the usual accompanying calls of 'How about it?' I actually broke the habit of an entire holiday and indicated that finally my answer was yes.

The floodgates opened, and on the bush telegraph (no pun) all manner of hell not only broke loose but went on a wild rampage. Thunderbirds are going!

I was ferried over to Monkey Island (25 minutes by jet ski) in a convoy of expectant dudes. I say convoy – it was practically a traffic jam. The sea speed record would definitely been broken on that day, such was the guys' collective excitement of finally nailing their quarry. In jungle speak this would be a prize kill after many fruitless safaris. It was a popular boat trip with the tourists, but as providence was shining brightly there were no scheduled excursions booked for that day.

I was getting relatively excited about what was to unfold. The only thing (it transpired) that was relative about the proceedings was that it was the mother and father of the most boring (and only) gang-bang of my life. It made me disinclined to ever repeat the experience and also inevitably gave me a jaundiced view of Malay men.

One would assume that being on a deserted island with all manner of flora and fauna, clear blue skies, natural waterfalls, cooling jungle vegetation and an attendance of chocolate coloured young bucks would be a recipe for a rip roaring time. Nope.

Of the baker's dozen that were participating, only one looked like he might give my 'mound of Venus' a bit of a going over. Nassim was somehow softer and more delicate with his touch than the other mongrels. While his compatriots were rinsing out the used condoms in the rock pool (for I was only carrying six prophylactics at the time) I had him to myself. We had moved to the peripheral shade of the cooling jungle since the midday sun and lack of any *real* excitement was sapping my will to live.

I can only describe Nassim's approach to my twat as being akin to a sinner's guarded approach to hell. A mongoose and a cobra would have been on more loving terms. He eyed it with such suspicion that I felt he had been fed a line that the interior of the cave would bite his tongue clean through. He seemed to make a brave mental executive decision and made the plunge of faith with his cute face into the unknown.

A homicidal maniac with a chainsaw would have felt nicer. I was about to tell dear Nassim not to bother when divine intervention prevailed. Saved by a primate! A curious cousin of *Homo erectus* came out of the jungle and looked dangerously as if he might want to get into the act. A monkey stopped the monkey business, and thank God for that. Bugger 'veni, vidi, vici' – I came, I saw and I realised that a cup of cocoa and a Snickers bar is where it's at. Eureka!

What's the next thing on the list of 'things to do before I die of ennui'?

Come on Baby, Light My Fire (Or At Least Make Me Smoulder)

'How old were you when you experienced your first orgasm with a man?'

Without having to pause and think I replied: 'That's easy, I was 33 and it was in this very brothel on April the second at approximately 7.30!'

'Come on, that defies credulity – 33, for goodness' sake! What was wrong with you woman? Frigid were you?'

I rounded on my interrogator like a black mamba and in my most imperious voice informed him: 'Actually there is no such thing as a frigid woman, only inept men, and in my considered opinion if the population of the world were reliant upon the female of the species achieving orgasm, planet earth would be mighty underpopulated – say a mere tenth of what we have now'.

'I think you need to seek help,' he retorted.

I longed to say 'At least I don't need to suck my own cock while receiving both nipple and anal torture.'

My inquisitor was actually a regular customer at the parlour in Potts Point, Sydney, and we all knew his exacting sexual predilections. He took for ever to come, and often this meant the poor lady he chose for the session would end up having to pay a fine for being late from the room. He was arrogant and opinionated and was unknowingly stirring up an angry hornets' nest. He was sitting in the opulent reception area talking to some of the other ladies, and this particular subject matter was steaming up our collective G-string.

'Look I can come if I wank, but you guys make such a pathetic cursory stab at it that it becomes a disappointing foregone conclusion. We actually begin to prefer the former,' I stated defensively.

'Yeah,' sneered Yvonne, 'how would you like it if we gave you a mandatory ten licks on the old fella and stopped just as it was getting interesting – you'd howl the place down.'

'Anyway,' he said turning to me 'who was it that broke your duck? Hung like a donkey, was he?'

'If you would care to look in that direction all will be revealed. He's a regular customer of mine and he's got an appointment with me at seven,' I replied in exasperation.

'I bet you 50 bucks he's an Aussie rules footie player. That's the kind of guy you'd go for.'

'You know, it will be an absolute *pleasure* to take it,' I beamed, 'and an apology from you.'

The door bell rang (or should I say *played*) to the tune of the Lone Ranger, and in walked my orgasmic saviour. Izumi, a diminutive Japanese businessman, was very shy and softly spoken. His dress style was the consummate 'salary man uniform' – dark, well-cut suit, shirt and tie. My style at the time was all leather and lace, rubber and chains. We made quite a pair.

I had never viewed Asian, and certainly not Japanese, men as being sexually attractive, but Izumi made me feel more wonderful than I had felt before or indeed since. Certainly he was very romantic – who could resist being serenaded (in heavily accented English) to the Elvis song, 'I can't herp fawring in ruv with you' while watching the lights of the Sydney Harbour Bridge? I was smitten. He was very attentive and would make outrageous gestures of love in the style of hiring entire suites of the most prestigious hotels (with city skyline or harbour views) and organising a sumptuous supper for me when he couldn't even be there himself. Then there was the sex. He made every previous lover seem distinctly parvenu. His mission was to please, and to extract as many climaxes as possible from my willing body before he would even consider having any direct pleasure for himself. This should be part of the national curriculum, and laws should be passed to ensure that this modus operani is compulsory.

The reason he made love this way was even more intriguing.

Many Asian men have heard tales and myths regarding 'Gaijin' and their huge cocks, and therefore feel deeply inadequate, so this was their way of not losing face. Well, it works for me. I was so crazy about him I very nearly immersed myself in the Buddhist Nicherin sect, of whom he was a follower and promoter. Tina Turner attended the 'meetings' whenever she was in Sydney. Aimlessly chanting 'Nam maya ho renge kyo' (even though I didn't know what it meant, and have never had a satisfactory explanation since) seemed a small price to pay for bonding with my little Nippon lover. Shame he was married with three kids – nothing is perfect in this life.

We had the most clement love affair until his wife realised something was afoot. She then informed his place of employment about this 'something' and his employer told *him* that this 'something' had to stop. He then was honour bound, in ritualistic Japanese style, to tell *my* employer that the relationship was over. (These Nips move in mysterious ways.) So eventually, after a lot of oriental convolution, my boss told *me* that the best thing to ever happen in my life (man-wise) was no more.

Later, when Izumi withstood my searing launch into an angry tirade and diatribe of epic proportions (known in football parlance as the hair-dryer treatment), he explained that this was the way a love affair (or its ending), was dealt with in 'the land of the rising bum'.

'I asked your boss to help you and encourage you, and show understanding if you were sad,' he said softly. This merely brought more hysterical sobbing from me. I keened with the sadness and pain of knowing that, not only was it over, but that he cared so much he wished me to suffer as little as possible. He was so beautiful even when he was dumping me.

I fear the Buddhist thing went out of the window and I reverted to the most appalling shallowness – I was not only losing the closest thing I had ever found to 'love', but losing the first man who had ever cracked it satisfaction-wise.

'If it took 33 years for just one man like that to come my way,' I thought, 'then I don't fancy the odds against it occurring for *another* 33.'

How loathe I was to let him go. I used every piece of feminine guile, I cajoled and coerced, I wooed him like the most lethal 'Venus flytrap'. I didn't fight fair – faint heart never won 'fair dinkum', the best lover in the world. He was powerless to resist and we limped along for a little longer. Then he saw his chance to escape my tenacious clutches. While I was on a holiday in England, he relocated to Osaka.

Even that didn't stop me. I tracked him down in Japan and he capitulated to my demands. I organised a week in Tokyo and he resolved to meet me there.

Enter one of 'God's little tricks' . . .

One week before my departure date I met the *second* man who had ever got me off the 'climax starting grid'. Kim Siew was a beautiful Chinese man from Malaysia and, like his father before him, was a professional gambler. Gambling and fornicating usually go hand-in-hand and I met him while finishing a shift at work. I instantly fell for him, too, and privately saw him every day before my journey to Japan. To have 'orgasm provider no 2' wave me off as I left Sydney for my reunion with 'orgasm provider no 1' was, frankly, as good as it gets. I felt sexually omnipotent. 'Jesus loves me, yes he does', I thought.

On arrival in Nipponland, God, who by this time must surely have taken his eye off the entire world just to concentrate on me, decided to deliver 'orgasm provider no 3' – Tetsuya. *Praise de Lawd!* From the sublime to the utterly ridiculous: the Bermuda triangle was closing in and I feasted, nay *gorged*, at the table of pleasure. A squirming moveable feast, a synchronicity or 'weirdness in the air' was occurring and I felt trapped and rapt in its maelstrom. Too much, too little, too late? Nah! Keep 'em comin' because I'm just getting started. And this late starter can get used to this. Hog heaven, here I come.

Tetsuya, luckily, was going to visit his parents in Kyoto, so this made my way clear to reunite with Izumi (my first, maybe not my last, but still my everything). God, warming to His theme of being an all-seeing all-knowing kind of guy, decided to move in for the jugular and sent a 'Monty Python' boot crashing on my much-pleasured head.

The phone trilled and I answered 'Moshi mosh', like the clever clogs that I am – expecting it to be Izumi.

'Guess who?' a voice said.

My heart rose and sank simultaneously. It was Kim, and he was waiting patiently in the foyer of my hotel. I told him to give me a minute and hoped that he wouldn't notice that the minute was fifteen. He had moved heaven, earth and even more (as in immigration, visa and banking services, not to mention compromising travel agent confidentiality). He decided that he couldn't be without me and broke every rule in the book to surprise me. *Surprise?* That would be a huge understatement. I believe that famous painting by Edvard Munch, The Scream, was closer to what I felt. Bollocks, bollocks bollocks.

If life hands you lemons then you have to make lemonade. There was nothing for it: my reunion with Izumi would have to have an extra place-setting. The phone made me jump again: 'Moshi moshi' I said listlessly. Izumi was also in the hotel foyer. 'Gee I'm a popular girl, this blonde is definitely having more fun at the moment,' I thought.

When a crisis is in full flow, one has to keep a clear head – and this was *not* the kind of head I had envisioned. I went downstairs to experience a cringe-making oriental farce. They both moved to greet me and practically collided with each other, such was their separate passion for me. Had this been a horror movie (and it bloody felt like it) the hands that were held to my face would have me peering through, barely able to watch the unfolding events. Instead a calm inscrutable voice sallied forth from my mouth and said: 'Izumi,Kim; Kim,Izumi'.

I felt angry to be caught in my treachery in the same way that a philandering man lashes out at the cuckolded female partner. I was annoyed with both of them for different reasons. I felt like lapsing into Negress speak: 'I don't see a ring on my finger, boyfriend.' It was beyond my control and I had a strained and muted dinner *à trois*. Both of my men looked confused while I airily tried to keep my panic and thoughts of 'God let the ground swallow me whole' to myself. A humdinger of a Kodak moment.

Poor Izumi continued to be honourable and paid for my extra interloper's meal. He politely bowed and bade us farewell. I never saw him again, and frankly I was not surprised.

How to deal with a broken heart while an ardent lover is at his most disgruntled best. Kim started acting up: after all, territorial rights a man understands. Even though I dismissed Izumi as being a mere friend he sensed the truth. Thanks to being sinistral (left handed) he picked up that feminine trait of intuition. Some trip it turned out to be. One lover lost for ever, one who looked as if he was on the way out and one (poor Tetsuya) who wondered why I was avoiding his calls. And that was my 'purple patch' of Asian orgasm providers. I fear that Holy Grail has not really been attained since – well, not so collectively.

My best mate Madge had to wait even longer for her knight in shining armour.

'You did say you were 33, didn't you?' she asked one day, as yet another of her temporary lovers failed to make the grade in the sack. She had just turned 38 and obviously used me as some kind of benchmark for the latest time that one should have to wait for a 'tongue-fu-king'.

'Yes, but don't worry, you'll get there in the end. You've only had a few hundred lovers – you've got to wade through another few billion or so to get results, but it will happen as sure as eggs are eggs,' I assured her none too convincingly.

'I'm beginning to think there's some thing wrong with my "box". Can you have a look at it for me?'

'No I bloody can't!' I laughed 'I'm your mate, not your gynaecologist.'

'Well, I can't seem to get any of these guys to go anywhere near it. I even had it all checked out at the clap clinic, just in case I was bunging out a strange aroma or something.'

'And did they keel over with their legs shaking up in the air?'

'Be serious,' she said, sounding despondent. 'There has to be a reason why nobody wants to munch my lunch.'

'Look,' I explained patiently. 'Men are bone idle when it comes to that, you've just had a run of bad luck – I told you before, there's no such thing as frigid . . .'

She interrupted me in full flow: 'Only inept men. How many times have I heard that?'

'Well it happens to be true. Why not just ask a prospective lover if he likes giving head?' I suggested. 'That way you don't have to wonder and you can stop worrying about it.'

'I'm just resigning my self to the shower nozzle and power tools from sex shops from now on. That's it for me, it's too disappointing.'

And that appeared to be that. However, along came 'Wot'. We christened him in this way because he was a gormless gobshite. He didn't fit the usual profile of being an executive booted-and-suited guy, which Madge usually favoured, but she had soldiered on with her quest and changed tack with 'a bit of rough'. He was as boring as a pneumatic drill and had the charisma of a brown dog, but he finally made my mate squeal with long awaited delight. Why? Because he wanted to please her and he persisted (boy did he have to work hard) until he got the desired result.

It really was (and is) that simple.

A man *always* comes. But for a woman, waiting for that elusive bliss is very tedious. Lazy lovers should be named and shamed or treated to the medieval pastime of dodging rotten cabbages while incarcerated in the stocks, or at the very least the water ducking machine. The amount of time I have devoted to making a man feel yummy is in stark contrast with those who have barely bothered to 'step up to the plate' at all.

We ladies have become adept at reading maps while in automotive motion, so telling you where to go and how to do it (cunnilingus-wise) is a piece of piss.

Come on you guys: *must try harder!*

Entente Cordiale (Kofi, We Need You)

'**D**o you mind if I'm black, because I don't want to get there and find that you don't see black people.

What a conundrum! I actually *did* mind but decided to err on the side of 'What the hell'.

Why was I being so appallingly politically incorrect? Because seeing a black man as a customer is totally different (nine times out of ten) to seeing a common-or-garden white Anglo-Saxon.

Also, life is too short to wonder whether or not one is going to a) get paid, b) get robbed or c) be treated with barely concealed distain. The years of Arthur Hailey's *Roots* have come back to bite the white man on his skinny arse. And after years of oppression who can blame them? I speak as I find, and I speak with great experience.

However, my fate was sealed and my colour bar was temporarily lifted. He came swaggering up the stairs, all baseball cap and stealth fighter trainers. How my heart sank.

'Well no wonder nobody wanted to point you in the direction of a public convenience,' I said as he came through my front door.

He had previously rung to say he was running late because he couldn't find a toilet (having travelled all the way from London). He complained that 'everyone was unfriendly'. I was not in the least surprised. He looked like a perfect mugger.

Never judge a book by its cover? This hard back (quarterback) was screaming Danger, Danger, Danger, Dive, Dive, Dive!

We did the usual 'How long did your journey take' – 'Lovely view you've got here', then attempted to get down to the business of 'how much for how long' They were prickly pleasantries exchanged with a deep feeling of suspicion on both sides. But there was a problem.

He appeared to have an inherent mistrust matched only by mine. I wanted my pecuniary advantages up front (which is not altogether an uncommon practice in the world of prostitution – in fact it's practically written into the constitution). He, on the other hand was so mightily tired of getting ripped off by white chicks that he was loathe to do so. Why, you might ask, would you go to see a lady when you felt from extensive experience that it would not pan out as the date of the century? Easy.

Black women (workers) wouldn't put up with their shit. A female negress once divulged to me this little secret: 'We let you white women deal with their sorry ass.' Meaning, of course, that they were (as a generality) a nightmare. So I had a sexual reject (from my black sister's point of view) standing over me asserting his unalienable right to a honkie sorting him out. This is a lot to present to a diminutive, untrusting hooker's door.

Stand off at the Okay Corral was in progress. In stature I was David to his goliath. He was all 6'2" of athlete (honed, I assumed, by running away from the cops). I was 5'2" of quivering jelly, though I inwardly congratulated myself on having the heaviest digital TV in the universe. ('Try grabbing *that* and legging it down the stairs,' I thought.)

I have heard that crapping in one's hand and slinging it at a would-be assailant was a favoured anti-rape/attack deterrent.

I was ready to do that in more ways than one. We locked eyeballs to see who would blink first. I won. I knew that he had travelled 60 miles with a hard on (and hopefully a wallet full of cash). He had chosen me from the images on my website and, since I bear a surprising passing resemblance to them, he would still have been game on. The rest was purely semantics.

I resolved to reward his faith in human nature with the going-over of his negroid life. He seemed rather pleased – in fact, *too* pleased. He had been so used to being disappointed and generally treated in a desultory manner, that actually receiving a good time was anathema to him. This to him did not compute.

'So you actually go into a situation *expecting* to have a bad time?' I asked with much amusement. He more or less answered yes, and said that since I was very lovely to him (which for him was a novel experience) he didn't know how to act and therefore felt strange.

If this is happening all over the world we are in a bit of a pickle, are we not?

Steve Biko, one of the original forerunners of 'black consciousness', made the comment at one of his many trials that the word black was pejorative, since it had come to be used, and seen, as a negative term – black sheep of the family, black economy, black mark against one's name and, of course, that old chestnut taught at the mother's knee, black bogeyman.

The same prejudices are levelled at prostitution. It's deemed to be a sad and negative term. Prostitute (and onomatopoeically it's such a harsh word, usually spat with venom) means to misguided minds promiscuous, untrustworthy, a woman of easy virtue, unclean, sad and, above all, somebody who deserves the approbation and denigration that is ultimately heaped upon her.

Well all I can say is, thank god for the unsung heroines of this world. No MBE or whatever gong the government routinely doles out for services to the public has ever, as far as I know, been presented to a sex worker. (I can just hear the Queen asking me 'and what do you do?')

And why not, pray? Are we not the glue that holds the fabric of society together? Unfaithful men are nicer to their partners (admittedly out of guilt). Captains of industry can think straight after an 'empty', and the socially dysfunctional feel less alienated by our care, understanding and kindness. We should be put on the payroll of all major corporations. It seems like the mother of all oversights. But then I would say that, wouldn't I?

Get your act together Tone, you can put on your pseudo 'estuary' voice and proclaim that your (imagined) party of the masses is finally recognising a body of people that have been vilified and castigated for too long.

Medals can be doled out retrospectively, and there will be a great march through London – which no man will attend because it would show his support and he would therefore be deemed guilty (by association) of 'fraternising with the slatterns'.

Churchill's 'never has so much been owed by so many to so few' seems fair comment. Why do the most magnificent body of women go unrecognised for what they do? Fuck political expediency. If every member of Parliament who has ever visited an escort stood up to be counted the charlady at Westminster could do a grand job of polishing the benches: I am assured there would not be too many bums on seats.

How come dinner ladies and lollypop men get all the fun when the medals of recognition are handed out? What I dish up is much tastier to the tonsils, and as for zebra crossings – *pah!* I lead them into temptation in much more fetching uniforms.

Judging people by their appearance or work title is ignorant. Whatever happened to the content of one's character?

Since my heavy metal days my mode of apparel has neatly segued into something more, shall we say, 'elegant chic' – though I'm still sometimes taken to task by dudes whose multi-pierced faces look like a hamster's playground.

A few years ago some scaffolders fell foul of my 'I'm as mad as hell and I'm not gonna take it any more' moments. I used to wear lots of leather and chains, not to express my sexual preference but as a way of asserting my right to individuality. Plus, when one is stage diving or moshing in the pit at rock gigs (as is my wont) one fits in with the surrounding head bangers. These building site morons thought it would be a chuckle to scream '*Whiplash!*' and '*Come on, whip me and fuck me!*' I rather took exception to their ridiculous jibes and, dumping my heavy bags of shopping on the ground, challenged them to a verbal duel.

Strangely nobody wanted to mess with this indignant leather-clad woman. Especially as I had the temerity to question the right to humiliate or intimidate, any woman passing by. (Eddie Izzard advanced the theory that those wandering in packs of five did so because they only had a fifth of a brain. Quite.)

This pathetic covert aggression has often been levelled at me for various reasons in my life, and I simply had to make a stand. No more Mister Nice Guy, and don't fuck with Mr Zero. I rang the number that was thoughtfully provided on their temporary erection and asked for the gaffer. I related as concisely and calmly as possible what had transpired, and demanded that he meet with me and order his (by now cowering) worm-like workmen, to face my wrath. I was going to give them a piece of my mind. Terry, the gaffer, did indeed assent to my demands and after listening to my story bellowed to his underlings to get their arses down to meet me. It was not a pretty sight: they were all swagger and snigger and frankly thought it was a bit of a lark.

'Would you like someone to say that to your girlfriend, your wife or mother?' I asked. 'How about your daughter?'

They got real cocky and bumptious and denied my claim. This incensed me so much I found my self saying, 'It's obvious to me that you're not taking me seriously, so when Terry here brings me a huge bouquet of flowers, the money for which will be deducted from your wages, I might feel that apologies have been made.'

Terry, bless him, told me immediately that this would be the case and to expect his flower laden arrival at my apartment the very next day.

Sorted. I would not take kindly to anyone punching me in the gut, and veiled insults are designed to do just as much.

The moral of these stories? Well, I had changed one person's mind and given a few others pause to reflect. How to change a person's perception? It's a rough road to hoe, but 'a journey of a thousand miles' and all that.

Our Tone has instigated entire wars based loosely on the premise of ultimately winning 'hearts and minds' – I admire his optimism.

Rump Wrangling (The Hard Yard)

While eating a very clement Sunday lunch, with an even more clement demigod of a man, (don't you get enough? I hear you cry), Mark, the owner of the Brighton Rocks, sidled up conspiratorially and proclaimed 'Hayden had his arse fucked for the first time last night, bless him.'

My magnificent lunch-date choked on his sirloin while I quizzed Mark for more salacious gossip. It was not meant to be a malicious aside or a carelessly thrown-away secret: this is the way we talk at my local hostelry.

'How has he got away with it for so long?' my hunk asked.

(Ironic that every man that sees *him* wants a piece of *his* arse – and I must say I don't mind 'rose leafing' him myself –. but I digress.)

Hayden put in an appearance a few minutes later and I asked him how he felt about 'losing his cherry,' at the somewhat late age of 26. He looked chuffed, and said he was sore but satisfied. My date had a look of incredulity, so I opined that gay men were not the only people that had anal sex.

Of course it's the thing that every bigoted dickhead thinks about when the word gay is mentioned, being as it is, an 'act against nature', but – and for entirely differing reasons – we women dip our pedicured tootsies in the 'bowl of buggering', too.

Women like it because it feels like the last bastion of abandonment. It also feels bestial, brutal and visceral. Women often say they like the concept of being raped (which confuses men and law courts greatly) and of being somehow 'taken'. Well, boy do we feel 'taken' when we have a great tool lodged up our 'gary'. It seems to epitomise the difference between the strength of men and women.

Years ago, in my love life, no man could get so much as a touch in that general area: it was a no-go zone, an abandoned goldmine with the words 'danger keep out' written in red paint. Now, for me, it's turned into a no 7 double-decker bus (please pay exact fare on entry). Nearly every woman that I have spoken to (quizzed) has said how fan-fucking-tastic 'it' was as well.

Every time a man went near my general no-go area (or, as I liked to call it, 'my Grade 2 listed building and object of preservation') I would try to deflect the unwanted attention by saying 'Perhaps you would like an object of a similar size to your dick rammed up you – after all, it's only fair.'

This was usually not well received, and the same old line (groan) would be volleyed by rote: 'Yeah, but you women love it.'

I assume that this precept is based upon the fact that women in porn movies appear to be having a spiffing time. A word in your shell-like, guys: she's being *paid* to look as if she is!

Men love (receiving) anal sex because all of their pleasure nerve endings are round the prostate, but where it gets confusing is when straight men (or those that proclaim they are) love a bit of a footle up there as well.

'I've never done this before,' customers (with an arse like jelly on springs) will exclaim.

But it's the men who are vehemently opposed to any stimulation even vaguely in that region who crack me up. Methinks that closet homosexuals do protest too much. Practising anal sex doesn't make you gay, just as strapping on a dildo doesn't make me a candidate for transgender realignment. Chicks with dicks.

Ah, now *there's* a complicated subject.

Meet the Lady Boys of Bangkok, the prostitutes of indeterminate gender at Boogie Street in Singapore. Male visitors are often warned to stay away, lest they 'get more than they bargained for'. And do they listen? Do they hell! It merely piques their interest.

In Penang, Malaysia, I met a kindred sprit of sorts. Dave was intent on spending every penny he owned to stop his philandering wife and her lover getting their hands on it. He was in bad shape – broken-hearted at losing his wife, and missing the children. He was also incensed by the fact that his best mate was living in the family home with the missus. We used to have 'rickshaw races' along Jalan sri Bahari after the Ship rock club had closed in the wee small hours. I would stagger to my two-pound-a-night hovel (having lost all my money in Australia), and he would go to the Chinatown part of Georgetown for a bit of 'how's your father'. I found him on Teluk Bahang beach one day, nursing a hangover and a secret which he longed to share.

He regaled me with the story of his last night's exploits: 'So I was standing against this wall, getting a top blow-job. Then I reached down to feel her tits, and . . . she didn't have any!'

'Flat chested, eh? I thought you liked mammoth mammaries.'

He shifted uncomfortably and sighed. He ran his hands through his hair (which is what most men do when they are nervous). Finally he said: 'Actually, all I could feel was hair.'

'What happened?'

'A sucks a suck isn't it? Doesn't make me gay, does it?' As an afterthought he added: 'God knows. I don't much like women at the moment, but I'm still a heterosexual man'.

A gay mate of mine, Archibald, said he could always rely upon getting 'sorted out' if he went to the sauna of *any* of the big seafront hotels in Brighton. The Grand and the Metropole, with their steady stream of business men, were a perfect hunting ground. Gay men have become bored with sex, he claims, if it always has to be with the same pool of available homosexuals. To 'convert' a straight man is deemed to be quite a feather in one's cap. Not for Archibald the stereotypical hunting grounds of the infamous 'bushes' and the designated cottaging sites. No siree, he had gone up market. He never failed.

There's a commonly posed question: 'What's the difference between gay and straight?' And the answer is: 'About half a pint of lager.'

Many has been the man who has found himself heading towards the bushes at Duke's Mound in Brighton when chucking out time at the clubs has resulted in failure to pull a willing chick. A no strings suck? No problem! Unfortunately no such area exists (as far as I know) for women to get their rocks off. This state of affairs should be rectified immediately. As for lesbians, I have a very illuminating tale to tell.

I worked in Sydney with a Teutonic German called Ingrid. She was the epitome of the Valkyrie. She was strong and beautiful and a radical, politically disposed lesbian, yet she worked as an 'entertainer' with me in Potts Point.

Why any one with a peanut allergy would gorge ten Snickers bars a night in itself intrigued my feeble logical mind. So how she engaged in sexual congress with the 'enemy' was beyond me. We lived on the same street, in the glorious neighbourhood of Elizabeth Bay.

'Why do you have your blinds down during the day?' I asked once, wondering if the strong sunlight affected her as it did my palatial seafront apartment.

She let me in on her secret of afternoon delight with (I

assumed) her many lesbian admirers. I asked if they knew what she did, but in truth the question was rhetorical – she would have been kicked, rather than licked to within an inch of her complicated life.

One day I saw her sitting on a bench gazing out to the splendid vista of Elizabeth Bay harbour. She looked pretty misery-stricken (some would say all 'fur traders' do), and with concern, I asked what the problem was. She seemed reluctant to return my stare, but when she finally looked up with tear-filled eyes, she said: 'I'm in love.'

'But that's terrific news,' I enthused. After all we're supposed to seek out love as if it were our entire *raison d'être*.

She held my benevolent gaze for a few seconds longer, seeming to be embarrassed. Oh dear. She couldn't possibly mean *me*, could she? She of all people knew that I was a fully paid up member of the life-long,-not-budging, not even mildly interested in experimenting hetero woman, and that 'beanie flicking,' (however wonderful when performed properly by a man) was not something that remotely enticed or titillated me. How might I extricate myself from this situation, without hurting her already unrequited feelings?

'You know . . .' I cleared my throat and steeled myself to disappoint her: 'I really like you, but we have no future . . .'

She leapt from the bench in irritation, but moments later crumpled back beside me.

'Well, come on and tell me woman. I've got a shift in an hours time and I haven't washed my hair. *Tell* me.'

'You know every time my blind was down I told you I was having sex?' she said.

'Yep.'

'Well I didn't lie . . . but it was *with a man*.'

'But you're a *lesbian*.'

'I know,' she said,' but I can't help it I've never felt this way in my life.'

'So it's still terrific. You may have switched horses midstream, but hey, that's what's so great about this crazy life. You never can predict what's around the corner.'

She looked at me in anguish.

'You don't understand,' she wept. 'I'll have to leave town – no, make that leave the country. My entire social life is centred round my lesbian community. I'll be ostracised or worse.'

I told her she could join the 'witless' protection programme, just to add a bit of levity to the sombre proceedings, but it failed to raise a smile. I then had the brilliant wheeze that she could have reconstructive surgery à la 'Day of the Jackal' – but this jocularity could not dent the impenetrable outer shell of ennui which she wore like a shield.

'When I am with him, and I nibble the edge of his lips, I think to myself 'If I have to die, this is how I want it to happen – just nuzzling his beautiful mouth,' she sniffed mournfully.

As words go, this sentence was among the romantic I had ever heard, though 'I have one week to live and am leaving you a million quid' comes a close second.

Nothing I said could stop her mental anguish and the outpouring of hysterical emotion. I now had 30 minutes to wash my hair and arrive in time for my shift.

'And just to make life really interesting,' she continued, 'I'm Jewish and he's a bloody Saudi Muslim'

I told her that nobody was perfect (as in the movie 'Some Like It Hot') and she then added the killer sentence: 'He's being hunted down by his government for being a dissident. We could be caught up in some kind of political fatwa.'

Now I am a woman of very simple tastes, and being hung, drawn and quartered by either the entire 'sisterhood of lezzers' for fraternising with the enemy or being murdered for being an adjunct to a Middle Eastern free-thinker was so complicated a prospect that I don't think I could posssibly have achieved a climax.

There's nothing straightforward in this life. Just when you think you have a handle on it – *Kerplunk!* Stuff happens that just makes you think: 'Is this a dreadful dream or am I going to wake up?'

Love. As my mother would say: 'It comes on like a dose of diarrhoea'. I think I have inherited her inimitable turn of phrase. We all have our bits and pieces – protuberances to stick in and orifices to accommodate, things to lick and suck and varying degrees of gender to do it. It's just like a sexual jigsaw puzzle, with pieces that can fit *anywhere*.

Sometimes I have found myself saying to a particularly handsome man: 'I'd love to fuck you.'

The smart-Alec, camp reply has often been: 'Sorry love, I don't think you can get yer clit up my arse'.

Very funny . . .

Charging Like a Wounded Bull

The John Lewis partnership had a catch phrase that said something along the lines of 'never knowingly undersold'. I was never quite sure what it meant. Did it mean 'We are charging you more for the privilege of shopping in one of our establishments, you silly elitist sod, you'? It still puzzles me to this day.

I once actually had phone cards printed with a cartoon drawing of two chimpanzees and the accompanying blurb 'If you pay peanuts you get monkeys'. My research had led me to believe that I was a tad more expensive than the going rate, but as a marketing strategy it went horribly wrong. Methinks I had unwittingly upset the sensibilities of the other hookers working in Brighton. They got jolly cross, and there was somewhat of a backlash. Harpies have feelings, too.

Only the other day I read somewhere, that the luxury goods industry is deemed to be the *second* oldest profession in the world. Thank God I beat a Hermes saddle or a Cartier fountain pen!

There is a famous quote about cynics 'knowing the price of everything and the value of nothing.' Since low costs and stupendous quality rarely jump into bed together, how can a price be put on a sexual service or the person providing it? What *is* the recommended retail price?

I once perused the website of a rather lovely young man called Alastair. He seemed like a nice boy. We emailed each other with a provisional booking (me paying him) in mind. Within days of my initial contact I saw, with horror, that his original price for an overnight stay had been hiked up by another hundred quid. I rang him and asked with much amusement: 'How much will it be by the time I meet you young man? Will it have gone up by another few hundred if I don't get my sexual skates on?'

He was charm and good manners personified, and in clipped, cut glass educated tones talked about 'the inelasticity of demand', and mooting Rolls Royce as an example of 'charging for consumer perception of quality'. (Take note – not all would-be hookers are ill educated). Clever kid, and in a way he was right, for compared to the other offering' on the site he was, bar one other, way and above the best. He was also (I later found) worth every penny, but nobody likes to be gazumped.

Years ago freshly laid farm eggs had a 'little lion' stamp of approval, denoting top quality in size, freshness and even colour. How can one do that to a 'prozzie'? Easy.

In Singapore, escort agencies grade their women a) b) c) and d). I once went there with a couple of younger workmates. We were tired of encountering (in Sydney) the same old faces, same old dicks and same piss-poor attitude. We decided to take a sojourn, and see if the sex industry was any more exotic in this strange land of no smoking and no chewing gum. We collectively went for a few 'job interviews' and realised that, were we to take appointments, we would be charging different rates.

Oh, the shame of being adjudged by a hatchet-faced Chinese woman to be a mere c) on the attractiveness Richter scale! Even though I knew why she had deemed my grade to be (in *my* eyes) so low, it still stung my pride. In China a woman over 20 is practically an old biddie, and the next step for a prostitute is to take the false teeth out and offer really yucky 'gum rubs' (and, yes, they *do* practise this over there). I was in my thirties, but even though, in time-honoured fashion, I knocked a decade from my age, she dumped me in the 'delete bin of life' and made me squirm with embarrassment. It's a funny thing: you are what people *say* you are. My confidence plummeted, and I even began acting like a c). Some people say I act like a 'c' all the time, but bollocks to that.

My travel companions garnered an a) and b) grade. Lucinda was blonde, young and pretty with milky alabaster orbs and therefore won the dubious distinction of a) status. White skin is revered in Asia, since it shows (in the suspicious Asian mind) that you haven't laboured in the fields like a poor coolie. Petra was the same age, but she was dark haired and sported a very healthy tan – almost a punishable offence, to the status-driven male Singaporean. Lee Kwon Yew, the eminent prime minister at the time, even instigated a scheme whereby like-educated and physically matched people could meet, marry and procreate to somehow build a superior super race. Sounded suspiciously Nazi to me.

So we sexual 'three amigos' would very often go out to work together in Singapore. Escorting jobs weren't easy since *all* unescorted white females were thought to be sex workers (for once they were actually right), and we had to bribe our way into most of the smart hotels, making us 30 Singaporean dollars in debt before we had met our appointment.

It *killed* me to think that for the same time and labour I would receive less money than my counterparts for my trouble. After all, I was the avowed 'yoda' of parlour girls in Sydney. No one during my tenure there earned as much money, either for myself or for the establishment, and I always wiped the floor financially with my present mates a) and b). I was in the top three list of 'producers and performers' at every one of the three places I worked. But here in over-airconditioned land, the axis of bullshit and deluded judgement had shifted. My ego was badly mauled, I felt devalued and discouraged from even trying to be a good companion. The working holiday didn't therefore work out.

At one establishment in Sydney there was actually a menu, including prices with the title 'Fantasy, Fetish and Floggings'. Naturally we all turned into supreme salespeople and suggested, ever so delicately, that unless the largest amount of money was proffered for the time, then the service would be proportionate to the price paid. Had we been restaurateurs, our patrons would have been made to gorge on lobster, oysters and tankers full of Cristal champagne. A standing prick is not only bereft of conscience but is extremely malleable, and when a man is so 'hot to trot' that he's at a breakneck gallop you can, by auto-suggestion, get him to give you practically the shirt off his back.

Yes, pricing a hooker is very complicated business. Too low, and the punters will think you are a duff shag; too high and they will think you 'have tickets on yourself', which in Aussie parlance means you are a stuck-up, snooty cow. The most surprising aspect, for me was that the 'little Aussie battler' with limited resources would often be the most generous, while the posh businessmen were like the proverbial 'nun's fun-run' – mega tight. I have even seen male drivers of Jaguars, Mercedes, 'rollers' and 'beamers' pick up 'skag heads' (in pursuit of their next fix) who looked decidedly the worse for wear, when obviously the punter *could* afford to dig deep: from a perverse sense of power, or degradation maybe, they patronised the lowest denominator. Go figure.

At least an Australian tips a lady if he has had a good time. In England – don't hold your breath. I put up a sign once which proclaimed 'Tipping is not a place in China'. The silence, as they say, was deafening.

There is also the 're-branding concept' which was explained to me by one of my favourite 'business associates'. As an example: a Mercedes car of indeterminate model was launched to much hype and fanfare in Germany, but nobody bought it. Step forward my Mr Big in the copywriting/advertising world. They withdrew the car for a few months, upped the price by a few grand, jigged around with the advertising and, bingo, come relaunch it *flew* off the production line.

Could the same thing happen in the sex market? I very much doubt it. If the price so much as moves in line with inflation, the fallout is so spectacular it simply isn't worth the aggravation.

'What, even to me?' they will cry when told of a modest increase.

Here follows a joke. A man meets an exceedingly good-looking woman on a train. After a while he propositions her and asks if she will sleep with him for £500. She agrees, and is flattered by his financial advances.

'How about if I give you 50p?' he asks.

'Certainly not,' she replies 'What kind of woman do you think I am?'

'That's a fact we have already established,' he says 'Now we're just quibbling over the price.'

Jennie, my cosmetic consultant, once asked me if I had a January sale, or indeed a 'happy hour' to drive willing victims into my arms. Frankly I think anyone who even attempts these marketing tricks make herself look like the worst kind of desperate twat.

There's an old Malaysian saying that goes: 'Water finds its own level'. So when customers ring to ask if I am free, my retort is always: 'No, I'm very expensive.'

Charity Chuffs

Sydney, Australia, and my befuddled memory (so many men; so few who can afford me) can't remember if the year was the bicentenary in honour of the intrepid pioneers who helped create all that was glorious in both the outback and the metropolis or if it was another war (Gulf War 1) when the boats came back relatively intact. All I know is that the bay in Woolloomooloo was rammed to the gills with battleships.

My goodness, what an awesome sight. These ships came from the four corners of the globe. Full of the world's finest (although I fear the Army and RAF might have something to say about that) they were festooned with lights and bunting to announce: THE FLEET'S IN – ANCHORS AWEIGH!

Out in woop-woop (the dreary suburbs), husbands, boyfriends, children, and neighbours were being collectively abandoned by the good womenfolk.They were on a mission. They had all seen 'An Officer and a Gentleman', and even though Richard Gere might not materialise in reality, they sensed that the 'target-rich environment' down by the harbour-side was ripe for the plucking – they were going to fuck a sailor. Notes along the lines of 'See ya tomorrow arvo' or 'Gone for a root' were placed less than lovingly on the Kelvinator, along with thoughtful plates full of vegemite sandwiches and maybe half a roasted 'chook'. Anyone who actually left a pavlova for dessert obviously knew they were in deep shit before the expedition had begun.

Meanwhile, deep in the netherworld of the city brothels, the workers girded up their loins and rubbed their hands with the expectation of a humongous payday. Every so often a situation presents itself which is 'manna from heaven'. This was a *lot* of man and, boy, were we excited!

The respective warships even organised a 'dial a date' service for those wishing to partake in a 'tour' of the vessels. The Japanese, strangely, were the least popular (don't mention the war), while the inmates of 'Big Mo', the illustrious USS Missouri, needed to call in reserves for the overwhelming demand. Obviously this 'dial a honey chile' was just a ruse to get laid, but certain standards had to be upheld. They had to be seen to be charm and courtesy personified, but everyone knew it was 'up periscopes' and 'big guns firing in the hold'.

Last minute preparations were made, with the Navy boys getting a certificate of 'land worthiness', checking on the eradication of any pesky rashes or discharges garnered from sin cities around the world. Conversely we had a refresher course, (from our in-house gynaecologist) on how to spot a manky tool. Sydney held it's breath for the onslaught.

And nothing happened! It was probably the quietest the brothel industry had been in years. All of the regulars stayed away, assuming we would be up to our tits in ocean-serving gits. They figured that *our* naval base (condoms not withstanding) would be full of discharged seamen.

Meanwhile, for those imperilled on the sea it was game on with knobs. There's a well-worn route from the docks to pussy – up McLeay Street and bearing right through to one of the dingiest thoroughfares in the world, Darling Hurst Road or, to be more precise, Kings Cross. It's full of winos, abbos and derros, the dispossessed and the most goddam awful clip/strip-joints in the titillation universe. The street hookers were skag-heads every one, and if they weren't, their general demeanour was still the same. They looked battered, bruised and stricken.

But the Navy boys simply didn't make it to the professionals. The resourceful Aussie sheilas were taking no prisoners. In fact, were they to fight wars *anywhere* in the world they would win. They literally set up road blocks and ambushed the poor fellas. These women stand for no nonsense: they might as well have given the boys in white and blue a 'fireman's lift' over their shoulders. The word 'no' would not have been an option. When you know you are going to be raped, you may as well lie back and accept the inevitable.

Back in the parlours the mood was as dark as a Nullaboor Aborigine. We comfort-ate our way through bowls of honeyed chicken and barbecued 'snags'. We also growled at any poor reprobate who happened to saunter through our doors, sailor or otherwise. We had been led to believe that our boat truly had come in, and we didn't take kindly to the 'scraps' that had escaped the amateurs' dragnet. Sailors may have a girl in every port, but they're also known to spend all their money on hookers once they've docked. These suburban interlopers had spoiled our party and our inalienable right.

'Bloody charity moles,' said Robbie in exasperation. 'I wouldn't *want* a bloke after they'd had a root with those filthy sheilas.'

'I traded in me Holden for a Toyota on the strength of this little exercise, and now I'm fucked,' whined another disgruntled worker.

Lots of ladies actually handed in their notice (as in got up and walked out the door) and applied to another parlour 'closer to the perceived action'. They found that it was no better anywhere else: everyone was 'hurting'.

Men have always been able to find someone (as in non-professional) willing to service them.

In my day it was a couple of Babychams and a bowl of stale peanuts, and one felt duty bound to comply with the unspoken deal. It's probably one of the reasons I've refused the offer of 'may I buy you a drink' for most of my life (with the exception of homosexuals, family members and blokes that I want to shag anyway). Guys seem to think that once you have accepted the offer of liquid refreshment, then a night of filth and naughtiness beckons. (I once even had a guy take the drink *back* after I made it clear that half a lager did not give him the right to sit next to me. What a buffoon.)

'I never have to pay for it,' they boast. Yeah, right. So dinner, movie, drinks, clubbing, (drugs?) and transport don't enter into the equation? And even if the little lady *does* acquiesce to pointing the penis at the pudenda, how does one get shot of them? When a man pays for a professional, the dosh is actually 'fuck off' money. It relieves them not only of a weighty matter in their testicles, but the guilt inherent in getting rid of the woman that has just performed it.

My mate Madge simply *never* puts her hand in her pocket when going out on a date. She is used to being treated like some china doll admired for its virginal beauty. The ultimate trophy for the arm of any man (what I term 'the crocodile handbag syndrome'), she figures that with the amount of money spent on lotions and potions, gym, hairdressing and general grooming she deserves to be 'spoilt'. She's been on more dates than I care to recall (so many men, so few orgasms), and even then she doesn't feel she should invite them to her inner sanctum just because they have pushed the culinary boat out with the finest food and champagne the world has to proffer.

Yes, she's wined, dined, but (lamentably for them) not automatically sixty-nined. They put her on the untouchable pedestal to such a degree that when they are eventually allowed to do a spot of beasting, they fail miserably in the sack. Perversely, those that do cut the mustard in bed are less than forthcoming with their money. As you can imagine, the man that said: 'But I've paid for dinner five times – I think *you* should foot the bill,' was given exceedingly short shrift. His visiting rights were withdrawn forthwith.

Meanwhile I get laid and paid, and since my patrons are well trained the experience is not entirely without supreme pleasure for moi.

And then there is Charlie (short for Charlotte). The woman has more sex appeal in her little finger than the entire porn industry. I have seen her covered in horseshit and paint (though not at the same time) and she still somehow looks adorable. She also has an insatiable sex drive, and any man lucky enough to have her gums round his plums truly knows the meaning of 'the best head in England'. While I may have to arm-wrestle Charlie for that particular title, I needn't worry about being usurped as the premiere sex worker in my neck of the woods.

'My parents are rather worried that I might try to emulate you in some way,' he told in amusement, 'because I told them how much I liked and respected you.'

I didn't take this as an insult, since working is a choice thing (for me), and anyway she's far too busy giving it away to all and sundry while becoming a rising star in the art world. She has one small flaw, however – she hasn't got used to the concept of 'condoms equals not having to worry about pregnancy'.

'Fuck me Charlie, not *again!*,' I stormed in mock-angry tones as she reluctantly told me she needed another abortion.

It's very difficult to speak with authority, or to give advice to a person 20 years younger than yourself, without sounding like a condescending and judgemental plonker. I think I just about managed it, but we played out the abortion scene a little more than was comfortable.

'Why do you insist on doing what you're doing? Is it because you subliminally want kids?' I asked one day.

'Not really, it's because they don't get the full pleasure with protection,' was her stark reply. 'I want them to really enjoy it.'

Not only did men not have to pay for her first class 'service', she was prepared to sacrifice her health for their ultimate pleasure. What an unselfish gal.

Our Charlie is top-posh totty and has always met and bedded a Tarquin or Gerard at some regimental do or other. They are mostly commissioned to protect and to serve by land, sea, and air, yet somehow, in their public school-educated mind, protection with a woman is anathema. They seem like utter shits.

We're all given 24 hours each day, and how we wish to spend that time is entirely for us to decide. So of the three 'man- eating musketeers' (Madge, Charlie and my good self), who is right and who is wrong?

The answer, of course, is none of us. We make our bed and lie on it. It's simply that I prefer it to be strewn with rose petals (thanks a pad-load, Alastair), crisp £50 notes (thanks patrons) and the detritus of discarded condom packets, for although my body is not a 'temple' (more an amusement park) I prefer to maintain a healthy status quo.

An ex-boyfriend who was having a tantrum, told me that I was doomed to be buried in a Y-shaped coffin. Sounds like fun to me.

Aroma Coma

'So you sucked my cock, but you wouldn't kiss me – what kind of fucked up logic is that! Would you care to explain?'

My combative interrogator was a customer who at first seemed pretty much a standard deal. As time wore on, what emerged was a prevailing attitude that was beginning to rankle. He had refused to 'go down on me' as his penalty-sin-bin, for my not being compliant in the snogging stakes. (I thought withholding sexual favours was the sole province of women.) I told him I'd let him know the reason for my reticence to swap spit when we had reached the end of (for me) our interminably awful session.

I hoped he wouldn't ask, since frankly what I had to say, no matter which way it was dressed up and garnished with flowing prose, was going to be offensive and humiliating. He insisted on knowing.

'The reason I gave you oral but refused to kiss you is because your prick smells marginally better than your breath. Frankly, your mouth smells like a bear's arse.'

He was not best pleased, but we exchanged empty rhetoric along the lines of 'See you again'.

'Not if I see you first,' I thought. That was the longest half hour of my life (except for extra time at the recent rugby world cup) and I programmed my phone to recognise his number so I didn't have to go through that misery again.

Why do some men insist on thinking that women have no sense of smell? I have even wondered whether they think a sex worker has lost the use of her olfactory glands along with her sense of decency or morals. Or perhaps they think she is so desperate she will accept *any* conditions of employment. An even more unpalatable reason could be that we are deemed (as a sub-species) to be so inured as not to require the accepted hygiene etiquette of consenting adults in an intimate situation. Well, for me that's: *Prostitute, not bloody destitute!*

But if this man was a dirty puddle, then Toby was a cesspool. For sheer putrification personified, Toby was the Superbowl, Olympics and any world cup rolled sweatily into one. A more revolting, retch-making sight would be hard to find – though daytime TV might be a close second.

He had primed me earlier, regarding the fact that he would be bringing a certificate of 'road worthiness' from his GP. This thoughtful gesture was due to the fact that he had an unsightly rash across his chest, and he wished to allay my fears. This information did not augur well. Alarm bells were shaking my solar plexus before we had even entered the 'amore-arena'. When he arrived I knew I was in deep shit Arkansas. He had a face that only a mother with a 'seeing eye dog' could love. – and orifices that only a frotting pot-bellied pig could find alluring.

One of my favourite comedy characters used to be Benny Hill's 'Halitosis Kid' – one 'Heeelllooo!' from the HK and the whole universe would keel over from the stench of the putrid greeting. When the certificate-laden Toby arrived, this was my world. I had an entire mother-fucking *three hours* to kill while inhabiting it.

Working by rote, the words flowed: 'May I get you a libation?' 'Yes it is lovely weather for this time of year, though the gardens do need the rain.' 'Did you travel far?' 'Yes, I believe your car will be safe there.' 'Yes, it is a lovely view.' 'Well, you don't want to visit a hovel now, do you?'

I wished my dear mother (who can talk for England) would materialise and keep him amused for an hour, maybe telling him about the last meal that she had (it feels like an hour when she's telling me, bless her). I had a word with myself and gave myself a good talking to: 'You're a *professional*. Get through this and reward yourself with yet another flagon of champers.'.

Now I know why people take drugs.

We languished on my luxurious leather couch, which handily was wipe-clean and therefore sweat-friendly. I dodged his clumsy lunges like a semi-professional fly half. He looked like a parboiled pig in knickers, and smelt like the dags from a sheep's arse. Oh yes, prostitution is so exotic.

There was one slight setback apart from the obvious: he was a *lovely* man.

Erudite and articulate, interesting, and with so much to say and so much from which I could learn– the problem being, that I had to withstand the most noxious smell from his mouth in order to hear these pearls of wisdom. This was some Faustian pact.

Thinking on my feet, as opposed to the *back* that most idiots think I work upon, I decided to draw the longest, soapiest gorgeous smelling bath in the history of a working woman in crisis. I made a mental note to incinerate the lathering sponge three seconds after departure – the complete fumigation of the apartment would have to take a tad longer.

It wasn't until he stripped (I had forgone my normal 'Let me undress you' service) that I saw the size of my dilemma. The roll-call of bodily war zones became all too apparent. Either I could feign a massive coronary seizure or I would have to be the first (only) person to tell him that he stank. Why do I get all the best jobs?

From the top, and in no particular order of merit, what awaited me was: Dog's breath; ingrained dirt; fungal rashes in the folds of his porcine physique; the kind of 'jap eye' dick that is never going to poke its smelly head through the clinically over-tight foreskin; more nappy rash and, as a finale (or final insult), toenails that could have had rows of runner beans, sweet peas and strawberries growing in the accumulated dirt nestling in his uncut talons. The *pièce de résistance* among this plethora of squalor was so impressive that I nearly gasped – testicles that were so enlarged with what I assume was elephantitis that it's a wonder he had waddled through my front door at all. They were the size of Hove cricket ground. Leg before wicket be buggered. More a balls before bails He could have been 'not out' for years. No cricket ball, no googly, no matter how cleverly delivered, could have permeated this mass. What Dickie Bird would have made of it would have been unprintable.

The *poor, poor man* (Toby, not dickie). I bit the bullet and told him I could do nothing for him.

'Has nobody ever cared enough about you to tell you these things?' I asked.

He started to cry. My attitude was just about to soften when stupidly (but predictably) he argued the many reasons why he was so rank, justifying his condition by absolving himself of any responsibility. After three hours he left, without me touching his disgusting body.

Obviously it's the fault, somewhere along the line, of a woman. Mother, sister, girlfriend or wife – these are the people who could have steered him in the right direction, even though the big bollocks would always have taken him 90 degrees off course.

Saturday night, and everyone gets lathered up and sprays an entire can of deodorant down their groin (apart from Toby) in the hope that someone might want to get up close and personal. Why is this not the case when going to see a lady of the night? It's not as if it's a surprise. I spend hours being in a constant state of readiness (a bit like a fireman, except that I don't lounge around all day watching porn).

'What do you do if they smell?' is a common question.

Nothing usually. Just like a waitress who has to deal with an obnoxious twit, I grin and bear it with fortitude, inwardly chanting the mantra 'This too must pass'. Nobody likes the bearer of bad tidings, and I don't like hospital food. Visiting a sex worker is a highly vulnerable and sensitive time for men, and to say: 'you reek' would not only confirm their suspicions that we are ill mannered, uneducated dolts, but would perhaps result in a lengthy court action for ABH. Anyway, I've smelt worse in a Safeway queue.

I was in bed one evening with a very lovely young man who was insisting we engage in my *least* favourite position, 'soixante neuf'. I call it 'the unspeakable in pursuit of the uneatable', though I feel sure that's what Oscar Wilde said about fox hunting. My young buck was taking it so seriously that I started giggling uncontrollably and somehow segued into telling a joke.

'It's *so* sad,' I cried, sobbing with laughter, 'Those poor people. What a tragedy!'

'What the fuck are you going on about?' he murmured as he continued his fruitless (for me) task.

'The Titanic. All those poor souls lost – what a terrible way to die.'

My young man turned round to face me, and asked why I had suddenly thought of that.

'Because the story is printed on the newspaper that's sticking out of your arse.'

He (eventually) saw the funny side. But I wasn't being so far fetched as to be surreal. I have seen the most revolting sights but feel it should be left to an expert in Tae Kwondo to alert a guy to the fact that a grey flannel dragged across the pertinent bits and pieces could make all the difference between success and failure with a member of the opposite sex.

I bet they'd tub-up for Pammie Anderson.

Date Bait

'You must get to see some strange people' is the traditional self-satisfied question asked by men who think they're an answer to my imagined cry in the darkness.

'At least you do some good – think of the number of rapes you stop' is another 'guaranteed-to-make-me-want-to-head-butt-and-knee-you-in-your-misinformed-balls' *stupid* pronouncement.

For the record, my customers are the most chivalrous, kind and respectful guys I have had the privilege to meet. It's the men *outside* my working life (in what's termed the real world) who give me the creeps.

A few years ago, while I was on a 'gap year or three', I decided to follow a girlfriend of mine into the murky world of dating, from a reputable national newspaper. She was dining out with different men from all over the country practically every night of the week. It sure cut down on her Asda bill. I was determined to get a slice of the action.

My first advert was rejected. I had used words which I thought might set me apart from all the 'GSOH' and 'friendship and maybe more' staid offerings. Yes siree, *my* men would sit up and take notice of my 'too clever by half' entry.

The deadline passed, and I prepared myself for a deluge of male companionship (and most certainly more). The ad wasn't there. I rang to enquire about the absence of what must have been the most outstanding piece of wit and repartee ever to grace a lonely-hearts, kindred-spirits, looking-for-a-no-strings-bunk-up column.

'You used the word "invertebrate", madam – we can't have that in a national newspaper.'

'Yet you allow the words "kinky" and "sexy",' I complained.

'You also used the words "libidinous" and "licentious". Also "intemperate". We can't use those either.'

Imploding with frustration, (you can't reason with the unreasonable) I coldly informed him that they were less suggestive than 'satyr and slave', but we had not bonded and I decided to make the bog-standard maximum 30 words as bland as I could, reasoning that I could always beguile my respondents with my charm, wit and gay repartee. After all, it was what I did for a living, so it would be like shooting fish in a barrel. Fun, here we come!

I whittled the 60 odd replies down to 30 and started to seriously wade through what was on offer.

I never once considered the fact that I was a stranger in paradise, and that this was an arena where the 'old hands' would have the advantage over me. What a sucker!

If a man is 'as ugly as a hatful of arseholes' (no photos being available), he learns to hone another skill – to have a certain timbre to the voice, for example, or to sound mellifluous and assured.

That's obviously what my first three dates counted on to get me to their dining table. Outside the restaurants, however, it was a different matter – there was no way in hell I was going to munch anything else. For 'attractive' read 'maybe before he was run over by a Mack truck and hit with a flying mallet'.

'You're *so* pretty', they exclaimed.

I strove to keep the answer 'At least I didn't lie' firmly in the back of my throat, along with my rising bile.

One actually cut to the chase, and after getting me to scald my mouth with a hastily gulped hot chocolate (this last of the big-time spenders was in a hurry), said he didn't need any more friends, so 'Hows about it?'

It's never really been one of my life's ambitions to sleep with someone who looks like a cross between a smurf and a womble, so I made my excuses and left.

I also made a mental note to obliterate from the list anyone who couldn't be reached after office hours or who only had a mobile phone as a contact number. I'm a quick study, and I was getting with the programme. These men were probably married and were preying on desperate women, or (because they were physically and socially dysfunctional) found this the only way they could get a date.

Some were great on the phone, but couldn't construct a sentence face to face. One plonker didn't show at all (bastard), and the rest looked like the defeated remnants of the Abyssinian army.

Only two stand out in my mind as noteworthy.

First, a bald-headed, leather-clad, muscle-bound, Yamaha bike-riding dude from Swindon. I decided to mix things up a little and gave him his brief. I wanted to reclaim my avowed position of control freak, and therefore told him how I wanted the date to pan out – before he had even arrived at my seafront apartment. Yes, I even threw caution to the wind in that respect, too. I was breaking all the rules. *Never* meet someone at home, the newspaper said. Well that's what they get for denying my right to use the words 'lascivious' and 'salacious': don't fence my vocabulary in.

I also had the last minute wheeze of forbidding him to speak to me once inside my door. He had his instructions, and when the doorbell went I nearly had a heart attack. This was exciting. He was magnificent – and only *mildly* too rough in dragging me by my pony tail into the boudoir. Afterwards, he growled: 'Make me a cuppa,' then took me for a ton-up on his brute of a bike. Great date. I shook all over for hours afterwards. I never saw him again.

Julian, on the other hand, was a very handsome fitness instructor. He had a thing about older ladies so, bingo, eyes down look in!

He pretty much broke my record for the number of orgasms achieved over a 24-hour period (not telling). And that was it. No romance, just matter of fact servicing. It was somehow rather sad and soulless.

I'm a game bird (I'm game, she said, so he shot her) and five years later tried the same experience, using the same newspaper, reasoning that I knew all the pitfalls and, in the words of the Who, 'won't get fooled again'.

How hilarious for me to re-encounter three of the most awful dates from all those years ago! They had mastered the art of voice impersonating. Did they think (hope) that in the intervening time premature senile dementia might have set in.

'But we met before,' I exclaimed.

'Oh did we?' they lied. Very funny.

I know revenge is supposed to be a dish best served cold, but lying in wait like a piranha, waiting for an unsuspecting fool to bleed twice in a decade, is stronging it a bit.

I even tried answering ads placed by the guys, though this was putting me behind the eight ball because of the control that was being relinquished.

One intrigued me, but I guessed these accomplished campaigners in the dating world would be adept at finding a catchy strap-line. 'Hermes scarf-wearing woman' was what he wanted, and I was not going to disappoint him.

I knew my wefts and weaves, my cashmere from my vicuna — hell, I even had a Jaeger or Pucci scarf gathering mothballs somewhere. Obviously he was looking for an elegant and sophisticated, gamine, Audrey Hepburn type. We could visit the Italian and French collections at European fashion shows in London, Paris, and Milan. I could help him replace divots at the Cartier invitation polo matches.

I resolved to get rid of my leather/rubber bondage gear and hide my Deep Purple and AC/DC records. This was not in an effort to sell a 'pig in a poke', but to give myself the best possible start with my new soulmate. (I could slowly reintroduce them later.)

He had described himself as handsome. All I can say is that he was visually dysmorphic. What he honestly saw when looking in the mirror, bore no relation, nay, was not on speaking terms *at all* with what anyone else would see. Great body but a 'rough head', as they say in Australia.

When finding love contacts from a newspaper there is a point, in the first five minutes of the date, at which you know that you've been the victim of such treachery and perfidy (in relation to their appearance) that you want to haul off and smash what's left of their lying face. And the personality that had so enraptured on the phone was actually the one being reflected by one's *own* effervescence. It's 'crash TV' at its most cringe-making.

It got worse. As for the scarf, he wanted someone who would take control, and he even started to drag my 'Noddy ladder' from the balcony, looking for suitable sites for me to tie him to the wall. He thought this was perfectly normal for a first encounter. What a dick.

All in all I found myself wanting to crawl back to *my* life again. There is so much more respect and affection in the world that I inhabit than the one lots of people are putting up and making do with. And its *real*. No pretence. What it is, is what it is. There's no labouring under the guise of it being something else, though some do try to 'cross-pollinate' and are indeed looking for a girl-friend rather than a compliant female. You can't sell or buy love. It simply isn't possible to buy an emotion – and since I've never taken ectasy I can't possibly comment.

'Yes,' I hear you cry, 'but what happens if you fall for a punter?'

That, dear friend, is when the universe tumbles and crashes around one's bejewelled ears. Read on . . .

Hoochie Momma

A ny woman who decides to enter the sex industry is on a hiding to nothing, if she thinks Richard Gere is coming to rescue her. And quite what one is being rescued *from* is (to me) perplexing. Is it a job or a calling (call of the wild)? Is it temporary or a vocation?

Let's face it, if you do *anything* enough times, it can pall, and you inevitably lust for pastures new and greener. As Led Zep said, 'The song remains the same', and so does the view, especially when performing fellatio (elephantine Toby being the exception).

Athletes hang up their spikes, waitresses serve their last plate and hookers swallow their last whatever.

Having taken a sojourn from time to time, I must say, leaving the industry for *love* is a crock of shit.

'Let me take you away from all this,' Peter said

Yes, I most certainly did have these words ring out in my shell-like. He asked me to marry him, too.

Off I trotted into the unknown (Cairns) to start a new life of blissful domesticity.

I met Peter 'on the job', and at that point 70 percent of my 'jerk-work mates' were also dating or living with punters. They say most people meet their intended at work, and in our case we knew what they were like in the sack from the get-go.

Peter had booked the top suite at the Boulevard Hotel in William Street, Sydney. He had also booked me. I don't know which was more expensive. We melted into each others arms and

I found myself telling him: 'Yes, I will stop working. Yes, I will follow you thousands of miles up the eastern seaboard of Australia. Yes, I will marry you.' The fact that I'd had a slut-full, gut-full of working and that he was one of the most beautiful men ever to have graced the cover of *Gun Monthly* made the decision dead easy.

He was due to start a boat journey from Sydney to Surfers Paradise the very next day, and we promised each other to meet there after one week. I struggled to keep going at my place of employment, but my heart wasn't in it. The most gorgeous man had made the supreme romantic gesture towards me and my heart belonged to him.

We were reunited after a few days and kept repeating protestations of love and soppiness to one another. Romance is great if you're on holiday and have plenty of money. One comment was rather jarring and portentous: 'You won't be able to buy so much champagne on my salary, baby girl.' Oh dear, was that reality insidiously ruining my dream?

So love can reign in shack or mansion can it? I did try to economise, and triumphantly showed him the bottle of Moet which was only 20 dollars rather than 45.

'That's the sort code,' he smiled benignly.

I refused to lose my dream and, pushing all the voices to the contrary into the back of my confused mind, I continued on my love odyssey.

I wound up my life in Sydney within days, and embarked on my adventure into the unknown. If you don't try you will never know – and I am *very* trying.

The esplanade in Cairns was where we choose our love nest (I insisted on a sea view: hang the expense), and while he went to work I dreamt up recipes for his homecoming meal. I was living the Stepford Wife ideal and sweating like a dinner lady. *It was unbelievably hot.* Humidity in these tropics was often 100 per cent, and in keeping with the economy drive we couldn't afford the air conditioning to be blasting out all day long. I knew what it was like to marinate pork fillets in XXXX beer and concoct some culinary marvel for dessert, only for my homecoming beloved to say 'I'm not really hungry'.

I knew what it was like for him to tell all and sundry that I was an ex 'worker', but he would omit the information that he was an ex 'punter'. Hmmmm.

I also knew what it was like to be in the path of a raging cyclone, to be without money, to read about local tourists being eaten by crocodiles and to feel less than enamoured with him as the months plodded on.

'You could start writing that book of yours,' he said accusingly. He bought me a voice-activated tape, but my voice couldn't make it spring to life.

I remember writing on a piece of paper 'Now that I've found you, what are we meant to say, and now we're together what games are we meant to play?'

They were not the words of a happy bunny. I had swapped the patronage of hundreds (thousands?) for one man, and I couldn't make the switch.

The bunny hopped back to Sydney. He followed. I started to work again, and naturally he was unhappy and started to imbibe a little too much of the amber fluid.

The end came when I arrived home at five a.m, after a gruelling 10-hour shift, to be confronted by a scene straight out of the Godfather. The bed was awash with blood. He had gotten so bladdered that he had fallen over and knocked half his teeth out.

'You'll be leaving in the morning, I expect' I dully stated as a matter of intent. He naturally thought I was kidding and the next day acted as if nothing was the matter. The fact that he looked like a mutant from the 'red-neck county' was lost on him.

There was no bitterness, and the only mildly nasty thing he said (men have always got to have the last shot across the bow) was: 'You're going to end up very alone.'

He was right, and thank God for that. If that saves me from enduring a drunkard for the rest of my life, I thought, then *great*.

The dream was over and I couldn't have been happier. He replaced me with indecent haste within 48 hours. It wasn't true and it wasn't love.

I have often opined that love is a myth perpetrated by the makers of Hallmark cards – people just get so caught up in loving the *idea* of love. The only healthy dose I want is of reality

Falling for a punter is indeed a tricky one. If its unrequited it's a real pisser. I know that when I have developed an unhealthy feeling of love (or is it lust?) towards a paying customer the answer is unpalatable. It can *never* work. Meeting in some twilight world, where the absence of arguments about domestic bills or indeed anything, is very appealing and appetising. It simply cannot convert to the world outside the bedroom. They are two separate compartments and should stay that way.

I am wise enough not to even try to make a customer conversion. I couldn't respect a man who thought it was okay for me to continue working, and I wouldn't be able to erase from my mind the way we met in the initial instance (once a punter always a punter). He would drag out the moody fact of my 'past life' with monotonous regularity; it would be an untenable situation.

He would also have to be rich.

What of the guys for whom I *have* fallen? They won't have noticed the film of sweat on my upper lip and back, combined with my talking gibberish while pouring bubbly into a coffee mug, simply because I can't concentrate when they are around. They also will never know the number of times I have masturbated, just thinking about them. It's my secret, and I would die of shame and humiliation if I blurted it out in a moment of insanity.

They most certainly have *not* known me say: 'Don't worry about the money, its on the house.' That would be the epitome of a give-away.

Stitch in Time

'**A**re you a breast or bum man?'
It's a rhetorical question I often ask my customers, so that I can better understand my fellow man.

It sates my enquiring mind, and makes me more of a budding amateur anthropologist. The answer given is the one expected. How predictable, and how wonderful, are men? Easy to read, easy to keep happy. A spot of oral (like a cuppa) first thing in the morning and last thing and night and they are yours (if you want them) for ever.

They pride themselves on being able to spot a fake breast, and crow with pleasure at being able to tell the exact cup size of a woman who may not even have a clue (Rigby and Peller fitting service notwithstanding) herself.

However they *claim* not to like silicone implants: 'Nice to look at but crap to touch,' apparently.

The disparity between what men like, and what women *think* they like has never been wider.

At one parlour in Sydney (seems like I've worked in *all* of them), there was not one woman who wasn't thinking of, recuperating from or wanting to add more plastic surgery. It was like a Christmas carol as homage to the scalpel. (Sing along to the tune of The First day of Christmas: 'Six breasts alifted, five fa-ace lifts, four liposuctions, three ears apinned, two noses broken and a minge that can cra-ack walnuts.'.

What was wrong with these women? If the customers couldn't tell the difference between a sex change and the rest of us (and to our collective glee, in one case, they couldn't), they sure wouldn't discern a millimetre change in the wall of the vagina hall.

The South American contingent used their annual holiday 'rest period' (or the time off that their dreadful controlling pimps allowed them), to have a bit of freshening/tightening up of the body or face. God knows, they needed it. They worked like women possessed, while their no-good sons of pampas riders, gambled and squired other women. I suppose a man has to pass the time of day while his 'bitch' is making money. They would restart another 'tour of booty duty' with canula marks all over their body. Mmmm, nice. Very alluring.

But I must say it was the Aussie women who were a law unto themselves. Bandages on the wounds, and full body 'corset', which was compulsory for the lypo'? No problem! The cobbers would just have to work round it. As that incomparable comedian Kevin bloody Wilson would say: 'Can I feel yer tits – or at least stroke yer scalded cat?' The answer from the working girl would be, 'Just have to find somethin' else to do mate, I'm in recovery.'

The brown elasticised gauze, with front and back openings, made the minges look like a McFurburger. Were they ever to introduce a specialist fantasy for getting down and dirty with intensive care patients they wouldn't need to look any further than this particular parlour.

'Ya know, you're almost perfect,' an Aussie punter told me.

'How do you figure that?'

'Well, ya have great tits, but ya arse is kinda big and yer thighs are like those wrestling sheilas – maybe if youse went on a diet, or even better, if you fucked me senseless after you finished yer shifts, ya might shift a bit a lard.'.

Yes well, thank you Mr Scientifically Worked-out Dietician! The deal is this: big tits, big arse. It's that simple.

All the money, time and, ultimately, *pain* these women endured was relative to how screwed up they were mentally.

In the same way that counsellors and psychologists or psychoanalysts are often desperately in need of help themselves, these ladies were mistakenly kow-towed by the tyranny of the beauty myth when what they really needed was a substantial attitude adjustment.

They were still awful, stand-offish and sneeringly full of superior swagger with the very clients that were helping them pay their medical bills. The men didn't necessarily want a beauty queen, they just wanted someone to be *nice* to them. You cant have an operation for 'nice'. You either are or you are *not*. In an intimate environment, men sense (like a dog senses fear) a woman 'going through the motions'. It's easy for a woman to make a great man feel small, but the supreme trick is for a woman to transfer that feeling of greatness to a small man.

All the plastic-fantastic surgery in the world won't achieve that. However, I did notice that when I had, shall we say, a little help with my lips the feedback was astounding. On a very basic level homo erectus wanted, and imagined, my engorged mouth round his tumescence. That's just nature – like a baboon showing its bottom to its mate. (If its red, apparently, you're 'in like flynn'.) So my enhanced pucker was like a red rag to the male bulls.

A long weekend in Barcelona a few years ago illustrated this very point. On the Ramblas there was (as there is in most European cities) a museum of erotic art. There were different rooms, bearing varying instruments of pain, pleasure, and sensuality; movies from different eras, art from different countries. I was the only woman in the place (hurrah!). The men went about their perusal with a great degree of furtiveness. It was hilarious to feel their sexual tension. Upon departure, I asked the curator what the most popular, sought after exhibit was.

'Pamela Anderson sucking Tommy Lee's cock' was the perhaps not surprising reply.

As I said before: Men – easy to read, easy to keep happy.

Taking It In The Mouth for Cash

The year was 1987, and the spectre of AIDS was dangling like the sword of Damocles over the livelihood of many parlours in Sydney. The owners eyed with resignation the suicide equivalent of Beachy Head around the cliffs of Bondi. This was serious stuff. Would the men stay away in droves, and would the silence be deafening?

First the main four parlours (there was really only four of note) had to come up with a strategy, but they didn't know whether to make a pre-emptive strike with regard to the 'safe sex' issue. I have always been deeply impressed by the Australians' attitude of 'if you're gonna do it, do it right', especially with regard to the testing of sex workers, and the responsible parlour owners, implemented house rules to ensure that these standards were indeed upheld. But nobody wanted to stick their head above the parapet and enforce a blanket ban on 'bare-back riding'.

A ridiculous situation arose, whereby it was *left up to the individual girls*. The comedic fallout was quite staggering. Some girls will and some won't (and we *would*), but would it be with or without? We all kept our decision to ourselves, though those who wanted to practise safe sex felt that those who didn't had an unfair advantage – and tried to prise the definitive answer from their workmates. There was mistrust and bullying from girls who before the catastrophe were a cabal of camaraderie. Then there was the punter himself.

Would he err on the side of conservatism? Would we have to put a plimsoll line down the middle of the brothel, to pair up the male and female protagonists 'for and against'? Festering fissures, what a mess!

A poor unsuspecting punter came wandering in one day, and we lined up à la Miss World, cattle market-style. The lady he chose took him upstairs: five minutes later they were both back.

'Bloke here says he doesn't want to wear a bloody rubber, and I do – so he's all yours,' she said, storming off.

We took our line-up positions again. He chose another lady: they were back within only two minutes. She was a safety girl. This charade was replicated a few times more before a spot of good sense prevailed.

The shift supervisor tried to bring some semblance of order to the situation.

'All right you girls, all those that don't mind a spot of uncovered cock, get in the lounge right *now*.'

Then another element reared its head: wounded pride.

'Well I'*m* not lining up. If he didn't pick me in the first place, why should I fuck him now?.No way. You can't make me.'

The supervisor couldn't (and we knew wouldn't) sack the lady in question, as so many paranoid girls were leaving the industry in droves. Finally she bellowed: '*Is there anybody that wants to sort out this bloody drongo?*'

He had to slink away before it got ugly.

This scenario was played out in so many parlours around Sydney that the 'big four' made condoms compulsory. That's when deep mistrust set in. Any one lady doing well with her earnings was deemed to be not only pulling a fast one, but pulling it right off. The punters 'put the bubble in' and informed ladies they saw of others who weren't 'playing the white man'. These accusations were usually false and malicious, and nobody was eveer sacked. The industry was in a state of sucks-and-fucks flux, and in more ways than one. – because now the punter *changed his sexual habits*.

Where before, the sexual larrikin would not consider a session to be complete without a good hard 'root', they almost to a man capitulated and went for an uncovered suck. The safe sex rule was for penetrative sex only. Oral was a grey area. We were kept informed by all the medical experts, and the findings were (and still are) that it was so low a risk as to be non existent, the only proviso concernning cuts or open wounds on the lips or gums.

So the punter neatly put the onus of responsibility onto the woman. Thanks for that. Selfish? Certainly.

Still the punters tried it on. It galled some of the girls that some absolute creeps offered five or ten dollars for unprotected sex (as if that was all our lives were worth). I reasoned once that we should charge extra for putting the condoms back *on* the more frightened punters, but it never caught on.

Then an even stranger thing happened. Being a working girl, came into its own, with the status of: 'best bet' where cleanliness was concerned. We suddenly enjoyed the reverse situation, and men were (rightly) perceiving us as less 'poxed up in the box', than our amateur counterparts. They swam towards the light and patronised us in their thousands.

Phew, panic over. I often wonder what happened to that poor bloke who walked up and down the stairs like a fiddler's elbow. It must have been one of the first times that we got to choose to refuse the punter.

Choose to refuse – now there's a concept.

A popular bit of sport in the parlours of Sydney was the 'Sorry love, you're not my type' game. Men who by virtue of having hit every branch falling out of the 'ugly tree' found this was the only way they could 'get back' at women who were for ever rejecting them. In their minds it levelled out the status quo.

Because the better brothels were most hospitable to potential punters, with movies, refreshments and the company of receptionists and supervisors in sumptuous waiting areas (I called them sheepdip holding pens), the mega ugly heads could have a fabulous night out free-gratis, with a bit of insulting behaviour thrown in. We would introduce ourselves to these ill-mannered mooses and they would affect a pose of studied indifference. A cursory glance of disdain would be shot in our direction and they would give their well rehearsed 'Sorry love' line, before they turned back to the eager-beaver shot of the 'bluey' upon which they were engrossed. They thought they were terribly clever. We decided to teach them a lesson.

The parlour owner had also bought an establishment on the opposite side of the road and was (unbeknown to the media or the men) turning it into one of Sydney's most stylish 'houses of pain'. Because the 'Saturday night sport' club obviously had a parlour 'map' which they could follow all around Sydney, they meandered across the road straight into our own little honey trap. Revenge had never tasted sweeter. First we started to leg it across the road (to much honking of horns, and cries of 'ow much?') We would then *reintroduce ourselves*, to looks of utter astonishment from the formerly self-satisfied idiots. They looked as if they were seeing double (ha, ha!), though one dick was so plastered that he picked a girl he had rejected five minutes earlier.

After a while we got bored with this, and upped the pranking anti. The decorative conversion to a house of Bondage and discipline was now complete, and we therefore organised for more of these poor unsuspecting dullards to be led straight to the number one dungeon – whereupon we would *lock* the 'padded cell' and put on the grossest sadomasochistic movie imaginable – gimp-balled slaves being buggered senseless by masked leather daddies. We figured it might make their ring-piece do the quick step. They shat themselves.

'That'll larn 'em,' as my grandmother used to say.

Shy and Retiring

'I'll still be able to visit you after you've given up working,' some idiotic and supremely insensitive punters murmur.

In the last few years I have had a newsagent, butcher, baker, and probably a candlestick maker move on to different pastures. I have never tracked them down to their new place of business and demanded that I should still be able to receive their original service.

If a customer (for whatever reason) decides not to visit me again I don't exactly get 'notice' and severance pay, and conversely I won't inform them of any impending departure. Each one thinks he is 'special', which is testament to the way I can make a man feel.

When I took a four-year break to be a 'greed is good', Gordon Gecko-type acolyte, I was assailed by arrogant customers who felt it was their God given right to come-a-callin' when ever they were in the neighbourhood.

'Thought I'd see how you were,',was the empty rhetoric they would use as an excuse for crashing in on my new world. They looked really satisfied with themselves as I ushered them into my living room. Just as they were about to make themselves comfortable on my resplendent sofa I would take them by surprise by asking: 'Would you mind giving me your address?' (I also employ this tactic with cold callers on the telephone.)

They would look at me as if I had completely lost the plot, and a look of incomprehension would slither across their confused face – until I had to put my case in the bluntest of terms. Sometimes with men you really do have to spell it out.

'Well, I just want you to know how it feels for me to ring *your* doorbell because I am 'just passing', I explained to the thoughtless miscreants. 'Maybe your wife or your girlfriend will be at home. I'm assuming you wouldn't like that very much, and I don't take kindly to you thinking it's okay to do it to me'

God forbid that I could actually have a social life or 'significant other'.

'Been doing this long?' I will sometimes be asked – the subtext being that one should get in, earn a bundle and run for the hills like a dog retreating from its own vomit. If I turn the question round to ask how long they have been in their present chosen field they get awfully defensive. What is it a working girl should be escaping from? It's neither illegal nor a danger to one's health (though I do get a bit of repetitive strain injury in certain parts of my anatomy). An athlete or sportsperson may have to retire due to not being able to compete at the highest level, but that doesn't apply in this exasperating netherworld. There would be no 'leaving do', with the presentation of a gold watch; no speeches made regarding my 'services to men'. Nothing. Just walk away whistling and run a B&B for the rest of my life? I think not.

My friends won't think less or more of me for changing jobs and I won't be a different person. Not for one second have I considered that working as I do in this industry precludes anyone respecting or liking me. Those that mind don't matter, and those that matter don't mind.

I have a wonderful photo which shows me flanked on one side by the fabulous Reverend Mary and on the other by a former mayoress of Brighton. What an unholy triumvirate we made! How did this come about? I 'did my bit for the community' in a slightly different way by attending and helping committee meetings for action and regeneration groups in my area. It was an insightful time meeting politicians, police, and council chiefs responsible for the area.

I was invited to a launch for a new informative tourist guide, where the great and the good quaffed champagne and sweating canapés. An inquisitive soul sidled up and made idle conversation, though her agenda was plain. She wanted to know who I was and what I did for a living. I have always thought these questions the height of rudeness (and *no*, its not a defence mechanism).

'So what do you do?' she beamed earnestly.

'The very best I can,' I beamed back

She looked mildly disconcerted but pressed on with her overpowering rudeness. I steeled myself to enjoy the moment where I told her my profession. Hovering on the periphery of this unfolding scene were a few mates who noted with amusement what was happening. With a deep breath I told her 'I'm actually an erotic service provider.'

Time stood still, and had it been a scene in a movie everyone would have suddenly stopped talking and glasses would have hung in suspended animation between sips and lips. The hunter was now the hunted, and I enjoyed the moment immensely – as I have on numerous other occasions.

The same question was posed at a Christmas party hosted by the delightful Kym and her 'hubba hubba hubba, have him stripped and sent to my tent' boyfriend Simon.

I don't know why they persist in issuing me with an invitation to these proceeding as there's always loads of screaming rug rats and cigarette smoke. Kids and coughing, children and choking: I abhor both. But I usually go, since K and S are among some of my favourite people on this crazy planet.

The question having been posed, I answered in my inimitable style. The poor lady spent the rest of the evening looking terribly worried and telling any body who cared to listen 'Guess what she told me – she can't be telling the truth, can she?'

I refuse to play the bearded lady

Well if all these people know the answer, why ask in the first place?

More often than not I baulk at invitations when I know that I will be an object of curiosity – a bit like Elephant Man, only marginally prettier – the host or hostess making sure that other invited guests know that a 'real live hooker' will be attending.

'I'm not bloody going,' I complained to a mate once. 'They just look at me and judge me as if I'm the bearded lady at a circus.' I was always loathe to be what I thought was 'the entertainment'.

'It's not Carnegie sodding Hall,' was his acerbic reply.

I don't need to seek out approval for what I do, and what people think doesn't pay my rent.

It will be a sad day for the men folk when I do glide or segue into another arena of endeavour. (Modest, moi?). But I will be easily and immediately replaced. Look what happened to some of the stars from Coronation Street. No one person is bigger than the programme.

Will I make more comebacks than Sinatra? I will do what I want and cease when I don't want to. It's called *choice*.

Cult of Personality

'**D**id you know that Julie Burchill has mentioned you in her autobiography,' a mate emailed.

'Does she speak fondly of me?' I replied.

I did indeed meet La Burchill some years ago, and we did indeed appear to get on. I have never tried to ingratiate myself with celebrities (but would certainly make an exception in the case of Keanu Reeves and Ian Thorpe) since I'm not star-struck — they defecate and urinate the same as anyone else.

This is what she wrote: 'I have been sexually shocked only once in the last seven years; when my friend ****** the dominatrix came back from a club toilet fussing about her complicated leather costume. "Girl it took me half an hour to get out of this thing and there wasn't even a man there to drink it".'

Yes she was quite correct: we probably *did* have a conversation along those lines. However, I really was only 'playing to the gallery', telling her what she wanted to hear – I don't like to disappoint my audience after all.

I knew I was right was the name of the book, the supreme irony in this case being that she was wildly off course in thinking I was a dominatrix. She could not have been more wrong. Yes I *can* turn my hand to anything (such as a proffered bottom), but I am in fact softness personified. I don't wake up to sweep hardened candle wax from my bedroom. It's a three-minute egg and bread soldiers for me.

Be that as it may, people refuse to accept the reality, since what is imagined seems much more interesting. Fifty percent of what you think you know, and the other fifty percent of what you *want* to know is the key to fascination.

I went to see Julie, and we picked up where we had left off some years earlier, sipping champagne and talking bollocks. Julie is a very political creature and so (too?) clever. We have lots in common, including a similar working class background, of which we are both proud. Hell, we've even shared the same GPs, though I wonder if her tits have been fondled in examination as many times as mine seem to have been. We swapped platitudes about seeing each other again in another seven years or so, since we reasoned that we didn't want to get fed up with one another. She is very candid, which is a quality I like, but I had one quality that she absolutely *despised*.

She cannot stand prostitutes – or should I say the profession itself. I had not realised her stand on this issue. I have read some of her remarkable columns, but it wasn't until she very kindly gave me the book of her Guardian columns that I realised how vehemently opposed she was to the very concept. She mentions it all the time, and is totally scathing about the entire premise of prostitution.

'You are damaging yourself – you *must* have been damaged when you weere younger,' she railed.

I didn't try to defend myself since she wouldn't have listened, though I *would* comment that there are few people in the universe fit to lick my family's shoe leather, such is my regard for them.

'Would you be happy for your daughter to be one?' she continued.

I just waited for the hurricane of hatred to blow itself out. I was not in the least insulted: these are her thoughts on the matter and that's that. I assume that every piece that she has written as a journalist has to be the truth, or at the very least to be well enough researched as to sidle up close to it. Julie's opinion wasn't unreasonable, since there are many examples of women being oppressed or being victims. But it isn't *me*. And trying to tell me that I am vulnerable and exploited is obviously, to my mind, ridiculous.

She has not walked 'in my moccasins' or skyscraper stilettos, so how can it be an informed opinion?

I once saw a postcard which showed a man carrying a placard stating 'I can save fallen women'. Another man responds: 'Can you save one for me?'

Wherever there is deemed to be a misfortunate who has to be saved from herself or other people, there is always some scumbag willing to kick the dog when it's down. Or, indeed, to exploit the snivelling cur.

This is where religion, cults, secret societies, gurus and charlatans (or bad men intent on further damaging the already damaged) can have a field day. People looking for an answer or seeking shelter versus professionals, sects and self-styled gurus with their 'Tell me about your childhood', or, 'By the way, would you like to join, and give us all your money?'

At first hand, or with considerable research, I know this, because 'I have been that soldier'.

When I worked for HMIT, (that's the dreaded tax office to the uninitiated), I resolved to leave before my brains were scrambled to souffle proportions. As Dame Edna would say, 'it could bore an arsehole in a wooden horse'. I answered an advert in *The Lady* magazine (which is still supposed to be the height of good form an sophistication), and in my desperation I applied for a job as an au pair in Altea, Costa Blanca. This experience has honed a rule of thumb which I have used to my advantage to this day: 'Never do anything from a position of weakness.'

I arrived at Alicante Airport to meet my new boss. Every penny I owned had been spent embarking upon this adventure, and my stipend for the week was to be one thousand pesetas – seven quid.

He fucked me within two hours of my arrival. Yes, I assented totally (he wasn't the worst-looking bloke in the world), but this was not what I had signed up for. Worse was to come. He started to pass me round among his ex-pat mates as if I was a bag of 'gobstoppers'. I wasn't then, and am still maybe not now, a domestic goddess (we all know in which direction I have moved), so it wasn't my ironing and brass rubbing skills they craved. I didn't like my situation and resolved to change it. I caught a train into Benidorm and went to one of the many 'English bars' that proliferated ine the town. I was fortunate enough to meet a gaggle of girls from 'sarf London'. They took me under their filthy-mouthed wing and helped me to find employment. My remit was cleaning apartments after the 'pigs in space' (a term used by cabin crew of charter class holidaymakers) had vacated. Then one evening they asked me to do 'overtime'.

It was a time after Franco, and things had loosened up- Girlie bars were springing up everywhere, and these London ladies moonlighted there to gird up and supplement their weekly earnings.

'Get yer kit on, blondie – yer on,' they informed me one night.

I shook like a leaf in a sirroco wind, knowing that somehow this was terribly wrong, but that circumstances dictated there was no choice.

We were picked up by a Starsky and Hutch look-alike character: a Spanish Huggy Bear and a neon baby-pink Cadillac (I am not making this up). I was being transported in a 'pimpmobile' into unknown territory, while the girls squabbled about sitting on the two battle-hardened Moroccan ladies' laps – on the grounds that they would most certainly have 'a rash in their gash'. This was all unknown and very strange for me. I could barely breathe, such was my terror. We arrived at a ranch on the edge of town, and were told to sit at the bar. I was so frightened – I couldn't speak

English, let alone Español. A greasy gringo approached me. I looked at him, and said the only Spanish words I knew: 'Una copa, por favor señor'.

It seemed to do the trick, and after a few of these I realised that I had earned more in an evening than a month slowly dying in the service of the government.

'You fucking stupid sod, what the hell is wrong wiv yer.'

This was what my workmates thought of me on the drive home. I hadn't come across with the goods, but because I was a 'new clit on the block' I had earned shitloads of money.

After a few more days I decided to escape and put the Spanish experience behind me. I stood on the highway and stupidly hitchhiked.

Guess what – the guy who offered me a lift wanted to fuck me. I was so tired of saying 'no' and I wanted to get back to 'old blighty'. Every 10 miles felt like 10 squillion, and then my old mate God put a spoke in the wheel of an agonised life. We broke down in Zaragossa. It was cold (November), and the replacement part for his bloody great Rolls-Royce was going to take another week to arrive. When life hands you lemons you'd better like bucket loads of lemonade, and I was fair choking on it.

When I finally made it back to England I resolved never to be in that kind of position again, but would search within *myself* – rather than join a church of whatever, or follow a guru.

No, I wouldn't give up all my worldly possessions and be a sex slave to a self appointed figure head. No, I wouldn't separate from or cease all contact with my family to be part of some shiny happy people group. No, I wouldn't hold my urine for 48 hours and tell strangers all of my fears and darkest secrets as a form of 'stripping away the layers,' so that I might be inducted into some bullshit group of people that would be so brainwashed they wouldn't be able to tell shit from shinola.

Talk about 'target marketing'. Paedophiles hang round in all of the places where they can covet what they see, political groups infiltrate universities so that they can insidiously twist the mega-impressionable mind. Children who have been abused, often end up swapping home for a carehome full of twisted sickos.

Then there is prostitution.

I worked in a place once, where it was *compulsory* to see a 'head doctor'. The monthly visits traumatised me to such a degree that I told the brothel to stick it. Unfortunately for them I knew my own mind. Don't mess with *my* belief systems! Psychoanalysts and psychiatrists? Fucked in the head. As a body of people, they are without doubt some of the sickest, and really need some serious help.

I was able to turn the tables once on a guy who had won the heart of (apart from myself) the most popular worker in the whole of Sydney – Olivia. If the Bhagwan Rajneesh and Maharichi yogi had coupled to make a child then this piece of dog doo-doo would have been 'it'. He was a an oleaginous little slimeball. My workmates called him 'Swami Sam' and I eventually called him 'Mystic Smeg'.

Though I was taking an extended vacation in far north Queensland, I kept up to speed with what was happening with my workmates in New South Wales. This creep had snared one of the most beautiful women ever to walk this planet, and it was the talk of the brothel. When I returned for another tour of duty, *she* was away, but the grotesque guru came to play in my parlour.

There was no way he could have known of my association with Olivia, and even though he didn't say who he was and whom he was bedding, I had the situation under control. Knowledge is power, and I knew *everything* about this stunted gnome. What fun! He started his spiritually tantalising routine, and I started an Oscar winning performance. I clutched my head and started to feign hyperventilation. He didn't have a guide-book from which he could refer, for this situation.

'I see bars and a big O,' I wailed, shaking (very convincingly) with terror.

He was hooked immediately, and his brown eyes bulged.

He was going to jail for smuggling into Australia more drugs than Glaxo Wellcome. The reason he embarked on such an idiotic venture was that Olivia wouldn't marry him unless he had a few quid in his pocket. I had him totally in my thrall.

I was the burning bush, the second coming and the parted Red Sea rolled into one. I had him on the ropes and didn't let him go. He paid for his time, and *begged* me to tell him how his life was going to pan out, and how I was so omnipresent – an all-seeing, all-knowing hooker.

I pointed to the 'scaramanga' mark on my body. It is literally an unformed nipple which, had these been the dark ages, would have seen me burned as a satanic witch at the stake. This 'follow me, I'm the pied piper' malarkey was a piece of piss. And that was what I told him to do for the rest of his life. 'You must drink your own urine,' I chanted in a trance-like state. 'Only then will you be able to escape your baleful star.'

Sod it, in getting someone to cleave to a made up belief system I was beginning to believe it myself!

The poor dolt must be sick to his gold-implanted back teeth of his daily libations. What a naughty girl I am, and how easy it is fuck with the mind.

Apart, that is, from mine.

Boys with Toys

My sister is a widow. No, Colin my brother-in-law is not deceased – he merely spends every available hour, and a not inconsiderable amount of moolah, on his passion . . . golf. I once went round 18 holes (titter ye not) on a wet, cold Sunday morning. No wonder Sis is content to baste the chicken, till he comes home for a late lunch. The club house drink could not come quick enough for me.

I was lucky to be allowed on to the course. I once bought Col a wildly expensive 'golfing outfit', which had to be returned to the gentlemen's outfitters because it did not pass the ridiculously stringent criteria. Somehow the club overlooked my scarlet and black spandex animal print cat suit.

Golfing has been described as: 'a good walk ruined'. My inappropriate footwear was in the same ruinous state. I realised that to have the correct apparel, golf clubs and all the other bits and pieces was prohibitively expensive. Along the way I asked what the strange pieces of apparatus with bristles were, as I had noticed them placed at regular intervals.

'They're to clean my balls,' he replied in a 'Don't you know anything?' way.

Seemed like a strange thing to do in the middle of a round, and also a bit too close to the ground to brush up the old testicles. Ah – *golf* balls.

Men, bless them, love their gadgets – and no more so than when it comes to sex paraphernalia. I have taken to hiding my 'apparatus', on the grounds that if you give a man a choice, he is instantly dissatisfied with the very thing that he is doing/having at that moment. If I am wearing 'hold up' stockings, why of course they want suspenders. Delicate diamante-encrusted G-strings have to be swapped for lacy cami-knickers, black satin for white lace and, strangely, stockings for *tights*. I have adopted the stance of: 'You'll have what you're given and like it.'

Years ago I made the monumental mistake of laying out my 'instruments' as a surgeon lines up his equipment. I thought it looked professional, and the customers were like excited kids. I had invested in several types of anal beads, in various lengths, colour and size. Anal beads work on the same principle as the old 'knotted hanky' trick. (No wonder mums advise their offspring to have a clean one, handily tucked in their knickers at all times).

I had intended for them to be used on the men – but no, I had not counted on man and his eternal quest to do something different. I begrudgingly allowed a smaller pink set to be inserted into my big bum. Once the session was over I looked everywhere for them but couldn't see where my customer had discarded them.

When he emerged from the bathroom, I said jokingly: 'Okay, I give up. Where have you hidden them?'

'Hidden what?'

'The anal beads.'

After a long pause he eventually said: 'I didn't take them out.'

If you've ever seen a flea-ridden dog trying to scratch its tail, that was me. My eyes went from clockwise, to anti clockwise and back again, searching desperately for the tip of an anal bead-looking iceberg, protruding from my rear end. My punter looked rather concerned, although, I thought, 'not concerned enough to bloody take it out after use'. He had a little look, but was more concerned about getting his kit on and running away from the scene of the crime. What a dereliction of duty. I couldn't seem to solve the mystery, and after a few bowel movements and an anal douche as a final flourish, I decided that it would just have to be put in the same mental basket as to where odd socks hide after being laundered.

On a personal note, I prefer a man attached to a dick and a face attached to a tongue. I'm rather old fashioned that way.

I have never asked my sister whether she uses any thing that requires batteries or mains in the bedroom, but were the answer to be an embarrassed 'yes' I'm sure it would end up looking nothing like the original purchase – at the very least it would have to be completely resprayed. That's because my dear brother-in-law is a conspicuous consumer of 'add ons'.

I remember when he was courting sis, and if memory serves me correctly he drove a Hillman Imp (or was it a Skoda?). Whatever, it was a sardine can on wheels. Those wheels, by the time Colin had finished, were adorned by top-of-the-range go-faster stripes, racing alloy spokes and numerous other accoutrements. By the time the steering wheel (fluffy covered), rollbars, fluffy dice (made that up), and every other inch of the tin 'rust bucket' had been transformed to his exacting standard, it was worth three times more (or rather, had *cost* him three times more) than the original auto.

Only last night I cautiously asked Sis whether there was 'any news on the 'c' front'. This is a secret code for the 'project that dare not speak its name'. Even my own mother, who is not backward in coming forward, rings me to discover the fate of this project, so sensitive is the issue. The convolution is due to the fact that for approximately seven years dear Colin has embarked upon what some people would say is a foolhardy exercise. He is having a 'kit car' built to his exacting specification. My sister is stoic about the amount of time and money spent on this male embarkation of lunacy. 'If it keeps him happy,' she will sigh. My mother dares not breathe a word, and the garage where it is to be housed has looked distinctly bare for – well, a very long while.

A mate of mine, having gone to my fridge for liquid refreshment, asked 'What's this button do?'

As the words 'Don't bloody touch' formed in my epiglottis, he pressed – and defrosted my fridge.

Men! Always fiddling with things they shouldn't – like your ring piece or the (sensitive) nipples after orgasm.

Strange that their enquiring fingers are reticent to venture towards an iron or a washing machine. Interestingly enough, men make great chefs, but more often than not, only so that their offerings can be devoured by an adoring public, which is far preferable to their being an unsung culinary hero at home. I guess that's why you can't keep them away from the barbecue.

Most of the men that I've seen (we are talking double digits here) own Nokia mobile phones, and my prurient interest in all things leads me to believe that this is because it has so many more technological features. Only the other evening my sister told me in a resigned voice that Colin had yet *another* mobile phone on the go, when he hadn't even finished paying the contract for his first or second. It seems that having got them, he was less than enchanted with their performance, and rejected them because they 'didn't do what they were supposed to do'.

I will take that on trust and continue to dispense the kind of service that is 'advertised on the tin' *I am shaking in my Jimmy Choos.*

And what, dear readers, of the missing anal beads? They were found, to much hilarity from my plumber Rene, in the wastepipe of my bathroom sink. All I could think to say in response was: 'I've no idea how they got there!'

You Take the High Road and I'll Take the Low Road (How Low Can You Go?)

If Great Britain were the female body, Land's End and John o' Groats would never get so much as a cursory glance, let alone a nuzzle of affection. Antarctica? Along with female septuagenarians, every one knows where it is, but no one wants to go there.

'Tits first, I'm not a tart,' we ladies would cry as yet another spotty oik attempted to stroke or (heaven forfend) penetrate what they perceive to be the (hole)y grail.

'Why don't you set up a love making academy?' many mates have asked. The reason, I guess, is that if someone isn't doing it innately then any thing else would be 'painting' – and not panting

– by numbers. Who wants to receive a look which says: 'Shut the fuck up, I know what I'm doing'?

I don't actually have a map of Great Britain to hand (Colin, my brother-in-law, thought the genitalia would be the Isle of Wight. Duh!) but I thought Milton Keynes or maybe Birmingham might be the numero uno-visited erogenous zone, with Hadrian's Wall in second place – the 'moreish mammaries'.

World travel has developed to such a degree, and so many adventurers are experiencing the more arcane parts of the world, yet English men still insist on jumping a flight to Amsterdam or Tenerife.

I have met couples that pore over travel brochures for months to decide where they might waste their meagre savings for the holiday of a wife-time. Pity they don't spend a fraction of that time discovering what *really* turns each others body on.

'I've never felt that way before,' my patrons whisper.

'You should get out more,' is my jaunty reply.

The reality is that no-one has *ever* touched them in the places that I have.

How many massage parlours have invitingly advertised their services along the lines of 'top to toe'. Yeah right, in and out the door before your cigarette has burned down more likely. For 'complete experience' read – hurry up, I'm tired. The men can get that at home. Both women and men are not getting the best out of each other.

What I suggest is this. (It may sting a bit but it will be worth it in the end). Cease all activity for one month. Then, when coupling recommences, no primary erogenous zones are to be allowed.

I'm not a motorist, but as an analogy, if the major motorways are closed down (complete with no greasy spoon services for 50 miles) then you have to navigate the B roads. Apply that notion to love-making. Drive down the routes less navigated. There may be some side roads or dirt tracks, that have not seen activity for many a moon. They may not be your quickest route, but it will be a sweet ride (unless you encounter a dead end). Stop to smell the roses, bluebells, forget-me-nots and primroses. What's the hurry? Stop and have a picnic even. The journey is much more enjoyable.

My mate Harry said to me the other day: 'You must be keeping the entire male escort industry in this country afloat.'

'Yes, and I've never had, or been offered, a head massage or a foot massage without having to ask,' I answered in aggrieved tones.

If a professional is not coming across with the goods, then we may as well put on our kabuki facepacks and Crabtree & Evelyn moisturising gel gloves, shut down, and forget about rapture. It's such bad form. I would rather have no fuck, than a bad one. As my dear mate Kym said (when talking about eating out): 'I'd rather cook for myself. It's better than what is presently on offer.'

Why is nobody seemingly getting what they want? My customers opine that I sate their senses and have awakened them to what love-making really is, but it's really not that hard for any one else to emulate. Maybe they can't be arsed.

'Tuning in to Radio 4' nipples-wise before literally trying to return to the womb simply doesn't do it anymore. It's a chore, not clever, and more painful than a migraine.

I met a fantastic porn star (top five in the country) a while back. 'When they shoot the lady sucking cock,' he told me, 'Us poor guys move so far up the bed, we have to do a re shoot.'

I asked why, and he just shook his head: 'They fucking hurt.'

The porn stars don't even know how to do it properly!

Get with the programme, ladies and gents. Forget your drink and your drugs, go forth and explore. You know where all the Meridians and charkas are, so check them out for goodness sake. Travel hopefully, circumnavigate the body with an inquisitive mind and you may find yourself truly *sucking* the marrow out of life.

Boring an Arsehole in a Wooden Horse

My apartment is located on the main bus route to (among other things) Beachy Head. It also receives 'paying guests' who exhibit the general demeanour of someone intent on catching that very bus. I do wish they'd cut me out of the equation. Spending time in this sort of company is like assenting to buckets of cold sick being pored over me, at regular intervals, for the duration of their 'stay'. No wonder they find themselves doling out fat wedges of dosh for a lady to be beguiling and pliant. They are, (for whatever reason), socially dysfunctional and have a most soporific effect upon me. The tariff should be doubled because of the excruciating boredom factor alone.

People often quiz/interrogate me about the kind of person I reject in the course of my working life. The criteria would be for the kind of person I would give a wide berth to in civvy street – people with a bad attitude, or in this case *no* attitude to speak of whatsoever.

'What if they're ugly?' they ask.

I am unaware of any service provider that turns its entrepreneurial back on cold cash owing to the aesthetic appeal of the customer. (Safeway would go bankrupt, and as for Infinity Foods, don't get me started). It has long been an observation of mine that the more expensive the car the plainer the man (though my gynaecologist in Sydney was the exception to the rule). At least these individuals recognise, deep in their warthog souls, that there needs to be a little bit of rejigging in the pulling-power department.

So some vacuous bints go for a flash ride – Ferraris, Lamborghinis, and even the most difficult ride of all (barring wheelchair-confined men with severe cerebral palsy) the totally un-negotiable Lotus Ellesse – and think that's okay. However, if the man has no substance charisma-wise, I'm sure the V.8, or whatever the engine size or 'grunt power' is, wouldn't be enough to hold the most shallow Bimbo's interest. They would find themselves thinking 'What can I do to get out of this asinine situation?' Well okay, they wouldn't think the word *asinine*, because it's generally not in the bint lexicon, but you get my drift. So a person/customer can be facially challenged and it matters not an iota to me.

The dear, departed Queen Mother said something along the lines of 'the contribution you make at a dinner table is the rent you pay for the seat'. How I agree. Nobody has the right to sit like (in my mother's words) 'Numbskull'.

I once met a man who was on the list of Britain's richest men. He was squiring a mate of mine, and she asked me to join them for an evening meal so that I could be 'quality control'. He looked like a pig in knickers (like most mega rich blokes do) and proceeded to ignore me – which made me feel as welcome as pork chop at a Jewish wedding. He was just plain monosyllabic and *rude*. I withstood this breathtaking lapse in manners until I reached my personal 'how much more can you take?' threshhold. I excused myself by saying, 'You either have nothing to say, or you can *think* of nothing to say, or you are so rich you can't be arsed. Either way, I'm off.'

There were lame protestations of: 'Oh no, don't go, yadda, yadda, yadda,' but I had reached my bullshit limit. A sad postscript to this tale is the fact that a newspaper reported his untimely death while travelling in his personal helicopter some months ago. I can only conclude that the 'copter, as a result of his taciturn manner, had *also* lost the will to live

This getting up and leaving is *not* a luxury that I can fall back on with a bona fide paying customer. So yes, you most certainly may be mega ugly as a hat full of arseholes, you may smell (but that can be fixed) – but what happens when you desperately need a personality transplant?

David Merrick (Elephant Man) was a grotesque, yet he had wit, charm and personality. He was embraced by London society because he was entertaining, learned and knowledgeable and because he knew that his physical appearance alone would not be enough. So he applied himself,using the tools (no pun) at his disposal, and won over an adoring audience.

A few weeks ago a new patron, who was booked in for a *four hour* session, came lumbering in exasperated fashion up my elegant staircase. His first (distinctly unfriendly) words were: 'Parking's a bloody nightmare. If I'd known it was going to be this bad I wouldn't have bloody come to Brighton.'

While I was coming to terms with his combative tones, he continued: 'I must be 15 minutes' walk away. I've just been round and round and round . . .'

At this point I called into play the 'tune out' button. Life's hard sometimes, but no harder to bear than when a moaning minnie has the talking stick. One feels like the steel ball being slammed from side to side in a game of pinball: it's an insidious form of assault and when it's with a patron there's no escape. Captive audience? Pah! It's like that medieval torture, the head vice.

My 'id' longed to say: 'Why don't you lighten up, you miserable git?'. I let the wind of woefulness blow itself out, and just as I was summoning the energy to launch a charm offensive of my own, he dropped in the very words that are music to my ears where thinking of running screaming into the tundra is concerned: 'I'm on anti-depressants.'

Great. I had four hours with a human being with not one redeeming quality. Not only could/would he not hold a civilized conversation, but he wouldn't be able to come very easily either. Bugger. 'You're a professional,' an inner voice whispered yet again, 'so be a professional for goodness sake!'

I have never been a: 'where do you live and what do you do?' kind of soul, but I acceded to the lowest common denominator of mutual banter.

It transpired that he was a chiropodist. What a combination. It begged the question – what came first, the chicken or the egg? His expertise on the subject new no bounds, and like a new-born baby he made faltering steps with his knowledge about his specialist subject.

He was still edgy and difficult, and he wished to progress to the bedroom phase. It really doesn't get any tougher than this. Once more into the B(r)eachy Head we go . . .

Emerging from this passage of time (which sapped my will to live and made me make a mental note of the local bus timetable) was, not a new, but a distinctly *different* man. He was telling jokes, and his entire countenance made him seem so much more attractive. My forbearance, patience and energy had finally transformed old happy bollocks. Myself, I was totally drained.

I have met customers like this before. It's an ordeal just to be in their presence, let alone to be a passion puppet.

I have met a few men from online dating agencies recently, who bear out the old chestnut that 'they're sicko's or saddo's'. They do the 'parking', 'boring monologue', indolent two-step, and wonder why it's so hard to get a date, much less get a right royal seeing to. People skills. So may people make no attempt to be effervescent and stimulating that I think a tax should be levied against them for being plain boring. People pay their council tax for fear of being evicted – well, these individuals should jolly well pull themselves up by their boot straps for fear that no-one in their right minds would want to have anything to do with them. I know some Tibetan monks wrap freezing cold sheets around themselves in order to show that the mastery of mind power (along with their body heat) can dry the dripping articles. They would have their Zen work cut out for them with this particular tribe. It's a perfect analogy: they (the prize bores) are like the cloying swirling mist in the dampest swamp, and as it gets into ones bones it makes you ache with pain.

I don't claim to be a laugh a minute, although all I have to do is get my kit off and some are convulsed with tearful mirth. But at least I *try*.

My first boyfriend invited me to a dire evening meal with his parents and a few of his neighbours.

'This is Dr Manual,' he said, trying to ease me into the stilted proceedings.

I was not adept at conversing with that many 'grown ups' so searched wildly in my lacklustre mind for something (witty) to say.

'I bet you do everything by hand,' was my clumsy contribution. I had not only tried to converse but had tried to be funny, too – with results that you can only imagine. But at least I ruddy well *tried*.

How dare people sit like a bowl of milk and expect things to happen.

Some online dating men say on their profile: 'Give us a ring and we'll sort something out' – and that's it. Yes siree, that will *really* flush them out! They're alone because they are boring. Red Adair never bored so much in his tenure as oil driller to the most needy of potentates. As Helen Keller said: 'Nothing comes from doing nothing' Well all of these potential online dates need to learn some people skills, and stop wittering on about 'I keep myself in shape and am *told* I have a great sense of humour'.

Says who? Let me be the judge of that, Gunga Din.

Since Brighton is where I currently live (though after this book hits the stands I may have to relocate – to Outer Mongolia) I'm obviously in the midst of, shall we say, a fair few gay men. It doesn't do much for my sex life: I couldn't get laid in a fit, though I don't wish to do a Jonnie Wilkinson conversion)

Ah, let me digress for a second. Dear Jonnie, world cup hero, *very* easy on the eye. The siren in me wants to lick the sweat of his exertions from every orifice – and yet . . . and yet . . . I have heard him being interviewed. I have the feeling that were I to wait like a Christmas turkey, if you know what I mean, I would be left wanting. Okay, so he strives for perfection, but he sounds, frankly, dull. As does another mega movie star I know. I won't mention his name, since lawsuits and being a tedious bore are commonplaces of his life. He doesn't hold a conversation: it's an *oration*. He doesn't talk *to* you, he talks *at* you. Boring.

But back to gay men in Brighton: they're usually good company, entertaining and witty. Yes, I know they can be bitchy, backstabbing, petulant girlies – but that's not the issue here. Whenever I have spent a clement period of time with a lovely intelligent gay man I have to say these words: 'You're not gay – you're just not trying hard enough.' And so it is.

Let's divide the world up into uproarious raconteurs and generally great company, and put the pub bores, the saddo's on dating sites and the men who, let's face it are empty shells who couldn't fascinate a fly into a geographic site where the two would never meet. In the blue corner, one would be breathless with the sheer richness of conversation, and in the other – who cares? Misery loves company, and if they are paying for it, higher rate tax should be levied.

Bores are the bain of my life and must be expunged. Men, whether they are customer or potential fodder for the social life of Letitcia, had better straighten up or ship out. Boredom doesn't get entry into this babe's bloomers.

Cum On, Feel the Noise

One of my favourite patrons is Reece, 'man of mystery'. Why mystery? Well, I never ask and he never tells. I joke with him that he's an international hit-man, and he plays along and never disabuses me of that far-fetched notion. He likes to be blindfolded and then have a feeling of *let the games commence* – with the breath, footsteps and the clinking of other people in the room.

Sometimes I'm at a loss as to who I can rope in to provide the extra frisson required, and sometimes I've strained the bounds of what Reece would find acceptable.

Friends, neighbours, and even a few relative strangers of each sex and varying sexual orientation have been press-ganged into service. Show me a person who can say no to me and I will cite the fact that I've been having an off-day in manipulation.

He will never know the celebrities who have tickled his testicles or mates who have poked and stroked his plonker. Well, I lie slightly. Après fab session, with great theatrical aplomb, I often reveal his temptress or tormenters. They can be either male or female, and he doesn't care. It's all about sensation.

But a few hired hands have left after providing the sounds to pique his pork prodder, while one most definitely did not want to be seen at all.

Derek is put on bird shit duty

I call him Vanilla Gorilla and don't even *try* to think about the reason for his soubriquet – for you will never get it.

I wanted to create the illusion of a femme fatale fluttering his fertile flute. By George, I succeeded! More perfume than worn by a Saudi prince,was liberally sprayed onto VG. There wasn't time to shave his entire body, so I dressed him in satin and gossamer silk.: tactile, soft and, most of all, feminine. VG rose, as it were, to the challenge. He was as good as any seasoned pro.

The problem was – what to do when the session had reached its natural conclusion. The British public would have had his nuts for cufflinks. I told him to wait in a spare room until Reece had showered and was ready to pay him. Yes, *pay*. I made Reece slip the filthy lucre under the door, while VG 'knocked in acknowledgement'.

Francis Ford Coppola, eat your heart out – a dirty, dastardly director (me) had pulled it off yet again.

In this particular case it was the *sound* of other people, but there are those who want to be *seen*. Humiliation at first hand is car crash TV at its finest.

Derek said he wanted to do my chores, or indeed anyone else's. I rang my neighbour Ken and asked if there was anything my temporary domestic slave could do.

'He can clean the bird shit off our patio if he likes,' was the reply, so bird shit was his remit. I imperiously commanded Derek to follow me to the lift in our apartment block, hoping against hope (knowing my luck) that Murphy's Law would not apply with regard to bumping into disapproving neighbours in the common areas. After all, a slave needs his goddess, to look and dress a little like one.

Ken entered into the spirit of things by coldly asking Bird Shit Man to follow him to the patio. Mr Olivier eat your heart out this time! Derek applied himself to the task while Ken and I sniggered in the other room. The things we do for a buck. We checked from time to time to see whether he was being conscientious in his duties, and I then went back into nasty, surly dominatrix mode and snarled: 'You will now follow mistress Letitcia back to her apartment!'

I opened a door and promptly walked into the broom cupboard. I had imbibed a champagne too many, due to the lateness of the hour, and my sense of direction along with regal sashaying on stilettos was buggered. Worse, Ken had bunged everything he could think of into the broom cupboard to create a good impression for his slave, and all the contents spewed onto my head.

We both stayed in character, but the illusion was lost – I had stilettos of clay after all. The contents of a broom cupboard had let 'light in on the magic'.

Then there are those that not only get a thrill from being seen but from being humiliated as well. Bill was his name, a big bear of a man, a former merchant seaman. He was a transvestite, and I somehow had to excel in cross-dressing mode to transform him into a plausible 'Jill'. It wasn't easy; in fact it was nigh on impossible – like knitting gravy. His request to be humiliated stumped me until my fertile imagination stumbled upon a cunning plan. I would send him out into the street begging, in his Jill gear.

'You have to walk along the road and concoct whatever bullshit story you can come up with,' I said with a hint of satisfaction, 'but you must come back with £10 or I won't let you through the door.'

He looked alarmed, and a negative response lingered in the air like a well urinated lamp post. But he thought better of it, and off he trotted.

'Stay within my sight,' I called to him from my balcony.

This was a delicious scenario, first because he looked (despite my painstaking efforts at making him up) like 'a bloke in a dress' and secondly because his gait was all 20 stones of a sailor's roll. The general public was giving him a wide berth, and I watched with childish glee as the entire promenade parted like the Dead Sea as this apparition came lumbering towards them in size 13 Dorothy shoes.

Then he disappeared, despite the fact that I had told him to stay within my sight. He had gone down to the lower promenade, which was where all the tossers, boozers and dispossessed hung out. *He was going to get slaughtered.* I started to panic, but the die was cast by old cleverbollocks me.

After quite some time I heard a sound which drove a dagger through my already palpitating heart. Police sirens and fire engines racing to the scene of some . . . accident? altercation? Murder?

'Oh paint me black and call me Bwana – then weigh down my balls with lead shot!' I thought.

I had gone too far. It had to happen: if you push the envelope it's going to tear, and this time it was ripped asunder. The door bell rang:

'Blimey,' I thought, 'that's what I call a rapid response.'

I wondered how many lesbian inmates would make me their bitch in prison – I was resigned to my fate.

But it was Bill, looking most triumphant. He had 'found' some money – £13.50 as I recall. So a word in the shell-like of the beggars of Brighton: don't sit looking so sad and pathetic. Just cross-dress. It's much more lucrative.

I could go on for ever with tales of derring do . . . but I will adhere to the old music hall adage: *Always leave them wanting more.*

The Rear End

Whenever I used to whinge to my mother that someone had let me down or failed to remember me in some way, she used to say: 'You won't have them to thank.' How right she was – a wise woman, my mum. Bearing this in mind, I would like to say to my head teacher (the one who said I would 'never amount to anything') and to some faceless tax officer (higher grade) who at my annual assessment said 'we are interested in winners here, not losers' the following.

The sun is shining and the seagulls are scudding across the cloudless blue sky. A panoramic view – along with a bottle of the finest champagne money can buy – awaits Letitcia as she glides on to her balcony whistling a tune and sets her hat at a jaunty angle.

The best revenge is living well . . .